## Comments on *Eating Well with Kidney*

'I was very impressed with the content of this book. The practical chapters I found very informative, and perhaps more importantly, easy to follow.'

*Laurence Spicer, London*

'I have thoroughly enjoyed reading this . . . the recipes especially suit those who work, where I have found recipes in other books take too long. The language is straightforward and understandable for those new to kidney disease and those who are more knowledgeable.'

*Lisa Brereton, London*

'I found the book very readable and I expect it to help meet patients' educational needs. It has been thoughtfully put together and contains some very useful information.'

*George Hartley, Chief Renal Dietitian, Freeman Hospital, Newcastle-upon-Tyne*

'An excellent book!'

*Louise Wells, Renal Dietetic Clinical Specialist, York University Hospitals NHS Trust*

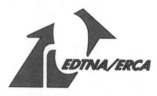

This book has been approved by EDTNA/ERCA
(the European Dialysis and Transplant Nurses' Association/
European Renal Care Association)

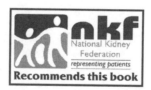

The National Kidney Federation (NKF) is a charity
representing all kidney patients in the United Kingdom, it is run
by kidney patients for kidney patients. The Federation campaigns
for increased renal provision and improved treatment. The charity also
provides national services to assist all kidney patients.

Publications recommended by the NKF have to be of a high standard
and easily readable, the recommendation is not given lightly and is highly
prized. The NKF recommendation of this book was made at the time of
its publication and has to be renewed at subsequent prints in order to
retain the NKF endorsement and recommendation. Further information
about the NKF and books it recommends can be found on its website
www.kidney.org.uk.

# Eating Well
# with
# Kidney Failure

*A practical guide and cookbook*

**Helena Jackson**, BSc, PgDip, MSc, RD
Specialist Dietitian, St George's Hospital, London

**Annie Cassidy**, BSc, PgDip, RD
Specialist Dietitian, St George's Hospital, London

**Gavin James**, BSc, MSc, RD
Clinical Services Manager,
St George's Hospital, London

CLASS PUBLISHING • LONDON

*Printing history*
First published 2006
Reprinted 2009 & 2015

The authors and publishers welcome feedback from the users of this book. Please contact the publishers.

**Class Health, The Exchange, Express Park, Bridgwater, TA6 4RR**
**Telephone: 01278 427800**
**Fax: 01278 421077 [International +4420]**
**email: post@class.co.uk**
**www.classhealth.co.uk**

The information presented in this book is accurate and current to the best of the authors' knowledge. The authors and publisher, however, make no guarantee as to, and assume no responsibility for, the correctness, sufficiency or completeness of such information or recommendation. The reader is advised to consult a doctor regarding all aspects of individual health care.

A CIP catalogue record for this book is available from the British Library

ISBN 13 9781859591161

ISBN 10 1859591167

10  9  8  7  6  5

Edited and indexed by Richenda Milton-Thompson

Illustrations by David Woodroffe

Designed and typeset by Martin Bristow

Printed and bound in Peterborough, England by www.printondemand-worldwide.com

# Contents

*This book is dedicated to all our patients –
past, present and future – and to the memory
of Lawrence, in the hope that it may answer
some of his questions.*

# Acknowledgements

Throughout the writing of this book we have been guided and supported by many people.

We are grateful to Richard Warner who initiated and believed in the task of publishing a cookbook for kidney patients, and to all the staff at Class Publishing for their help over the past few years. At the other end of the process we have been fortunate in our editor, Richenda Milton-Thompson who has contributed so much to the finished product.

We have been lucky to have a number of expert healthcare professionals and advisors who helped by reviewing the manuscript. We would like to thank the following for their comments and contribution to the book: Gemma Bircher, Barbara Engel, George Hartley, Sam Kanisius, Althea Mahon, Andy Stein, Louise Wells and Janet Wild.

We are also very grateful to the following patients, relatives and friends who brought the unique insights of personal experience: Lisa Brereton, Angela Dennis, Deryk Draughn, Lisa Mairs, Andrew Roberts, Laurence Spicer, Michael Watts and Norma Watts.

We greatly appreciate the help and support of our renal and dietetic colleagues at St George's and King's College Hospitals and the invaluable experience in meeting, learning from and working with kidney patients at both hospitals.

Last, but not least, a particular and heartfelt thanks to our friends and families for their love, help and support. With patience, enthusiasm and fortitude, they have tasted multiple versions of our chosen (and rejected) dishes, completed all those chores left undone and, uncomplaining, allowed a rival, 'The Book', to take much of our time and attention.

Helena Jackson
Annie Cassidy
Gavin James

# Foreword

Food is not only a basic need but also an important part of most peoples' daily enjoyment. Unfortunately renal failure can change this for the person affected as well as for their family and friends. Having to take on board new dietary guidelines and cooking methods can make daily meals, eating out and entertaining increasingly difficult to cope with.

The bookshelves are stacked full of recipe books and tips for various diets but there are limited resources for a person with renal failure. Dietitians are skilled in giving practical advice but they cannot be available in the home to answer questions and give cooking ideas 24 hours a day. There is an obvious need for more information to be at hand.

After 18 years of working in the renal field I warmly welcome this book as a valuable tool for dietitians and people with renal failure alike. I think it will make a huge contribution to the quality of life of many people presently struggling with complex dietary restrictions.

*Gemma Bircher* BSc, PgDip, Msc, RD
*Past president of EDTNA/ERCA*
*(European Dialysis and Transplant*
*Nurses Association/European*
*Renal Care Association)*

# Introduction

This book is about food and drink and kidney failure. It is full of quick, simple and great-tasting recipes for people with kidney disease, along with their friends and families. It is intended for adults at all stages of kidney failure, from those whose kidneys are working slightly below their normal level to those whose kidneys have failed altogether and who are reliant on dialysis.

Many people with kidney failure, especially those on dialysis, will have the opportunity to discuss what they eat with a specialist kidney dietitian. This book is not designed to replace this essential personal advice. Rather, it aims to help you understand the importance of eating well. This way, you can be better informed when you see your dietitian and other health professionals. We hope that it will answer some questions that you may not think of or have time to ask in clinic, and that it will continue to provide you with additional information and support.

The book is divided into two sections. The first gives some factual information about food and nutrition, with particular relevance to kidney disease. The second includes over 50 delicious recipes to show you that eating can still be pleasurable. There are hints and tips on choosing and eating meals, including takeaways, pre-packaged meals and food for celebrations and special occasions.

As well as being tasty and simple to produce, the recipes have been chosen to help you understand how to adapt favourite recipes and make them suitable for your special diet. They have all been tried and tested, and the finished dishes have been tasted by our friends, relatives, colleagues and patients. We are grateful for the help of all our 'tasters' in producing the end result.

Not everyone with kidney failure will need to make drastic changes to what they eat. Reading this book will reassure some of you that your diet is fine as it is. Most people will find they need to make only small changes to the way they eat. A few readers, however, may need to make significant changes, usually because of more severe kidney failure or other health problems.

Weight loss and malnutrition can be a particular problem for some patients with kidney failure. We hope that the recipes in this book will help those for whom this is a concern.

We have based this book on our experience as people who enjoy food and as dietitians working with people who have kidney failure. We hope that it will help you take control of this important aspect of your life, giving you suggestions for using food in a way that combines health and enjoyment.

# Part 1 – FOOD FACTS

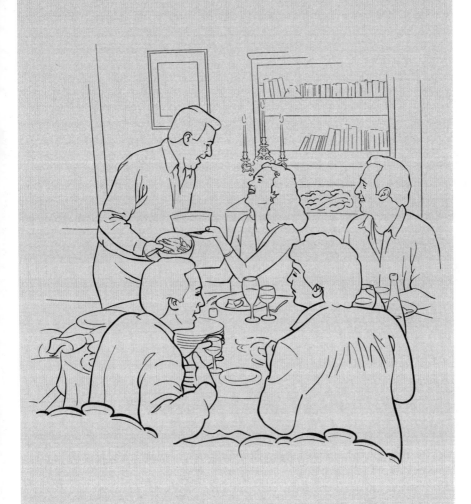

# 1
# How does kidney failure change what you should eat?

There is no single diet for people with kidney failure. Every one of you will have different medical problems and individual tastes in food that make you unique. The level at which the kidneys function, and the speed at which they fail, varies enormously between people. For some, there comes a time when their kidney function is so poor that dialysis or a kidney transplant is needed. While this book has been written for people at all stages of kidney failure, people who have a successful kidney transplant may not need to follow all the advice it contains as they can usually eat without too many restrictions.

The need to change what you eat when your kidneys fail is linked to what your kidneys normally do. Healthy kidneys control the level of chemicals and water in the body. Some chemicals are waste products; others are minerals such as potassium, sodium and phosphate which are vital for life. When your kidneys fail, the waste products build up and can cause symptoms such as a reduced appetite and weight loss. At the same time, the balance of some minerals and other nutrients may be disturbed, causing them to rise or fall outside the levels required for health. As these substances come from the food you eat, you may need to change your diet to control their levels within your body. It is also important to continue to eat a well-balanced diet.

Dialysis is a treatment that cleans your body of waste products, excess minerals and water – something healthy kidneys would normally do. There are two main forms of dialysis, haemodialysis and peritoneal dialysis. Haemodialysis involves using a machine to clean the blood for about three or four hours every two or three days. Waste products and fluid build up between haemodialysis sessions. To limit this build-up, it is important to eat and drink the right things in the right amounts. This will prevent unpleasant symptoms and side effects between dialysis sessions.

Peritoneal dialysis, on the other hand, provides a more continuous form of dialysis. This avoids the problem of build-up between sessions. However, some restrictions on what you eat may still be necessary. Unfortunately, neither type of dialysis is as effective as normal kidneys at balancing all the substances in the body.

Kidney failure and dialysis affect different people in different ways. Some people have almost no symptoms, others feel unwell from an early stage. Those people who do suffer from symptoms often find these affect their ability and desire to eat. Symptoms can range from being tired and finding it difficult to cook after a day's work, to experiencing severe fatigue, taste changes and sickness. This can lead to weight loss and malnutrition.

In addition, some people will have to restrict some types of food and drink although others may continue to eat normally. It is important for everyone to discuss their condition and symptoms with their doctor and dietitian.

A dietitian is an expert in nutrition, and renal dietitians have additional training and experience involving work with people with kidney failure. Not everyone who is diagnosed with kidney failure will automatically see a renal dietitian, but anyone who has difficulties eating enough, or needs to change their diet, should. In practice, most people who are on dialysis or aware that they will need dialysis in the future should expect to see a renal dietitian regularly to discuss all aspects of their diet.

A dietitian will advise on three main aspects:

- A healthy diet (a well-balanced diet) that contains all the nutrients the body needs;

- Ways of preventing – or addressing – any unintentional weight loss or malnutrition;

- The best foods to eat to control the build-up of waste products in the body.

So, almost every aspect of the diet can be affected by having kidney failure. Sometimes people find that the advice they receive is different from information they have been given about diet for other conditions (such as diabetes and heart disease). At other times, the advice seems to be constantly changing, usually in response to changes in their condition or treatment. This is why it is important for you to discuss any concerns with your dietitian, and ask him or her to explain the reasons behind any changes to your diet. You are an individual with your own dietary needs and preferences that are different from anyone else's. You may have other additional religious, social, medical or dietary requirements that affect the foods that you can choose. These should all be taken into consideration if you need to change your diet.

# 2
# Energy

## WHAT IS IT?

Everyone needs an adequate supply of energy for the body to function normally, for growth and replacement of tissue as well as any physical activity. If your weight is to be stable over time, your energy levels must be in balance, that is:

*Energy taken in (as food or drink)* = *Energy used up (by activity/exercise)*

If you do not eat enough energy, your body will start to use up its reserve stores of fat or muscle. This will lead to weight loss and muscle wasting. On the other hand, if you eat more energy than your body needs, you will become overweight.

## WHAT HAPPENS IN KIDNEY FAILURE?

Having kidney failure does not necessarily change the amount of energy you need. This depends on how active you are, as well as on whether you have any other medical conditions. However, kidney disease can make it more difficult to eat enough food to give you the energy you need. This can be for a number of reasons. Some people tend to feel more tired, nauseous and unwell or just less hungry. Shopping for food and cooking, along with other daily chores, can become more difficult. Lack of food can lead to weight loss, malnutrition and and muscle wasting, making it harder for the body to fight off infection. If you feel that you are having trouble eating enough, or are losing weight without meaning to, you should ask to see a dietitian. It is always better to try to prevent weight loss in the first place.

On the other hand, you may feel that you are overweight. If this is the case, your health may be improved by losing some weight, especially in the early stages of kidney failure. If you have more advanced renal failure, are on dialysis or are following other dietary restrictions you should also seek advice before trying to lose weight. (See Chapter 8 for more information on weight control.)

## ENERGY ON HAEMODIALYSIS

In theory, people on haemodialysis do not generally need extra energy. In fact they may need less energy if they are elderly or not as active as they once were. Even so they often struggle to eat enough, leading to loss of weight, as described above.

## ENERGY ON PERITONEAL DIALYSIS

Peritoneal dialysis is not thought to affect the amount of energy you need. However, people on peritoneal dialysis have an additional source of energy. The fluid in some peritoneal dialysis bags contains sugar and some of this is absorbed directly by the body while the fluid is in the abdomen. The 'stronger' the bag, the more sugar it contains and the more that will be absorbed. This can cause some people to gain more 'flesh' weight than they should. If you have diabetes, the sugar that is absorbed can affect your blood sugar control, which means that treatment will need to be monitored with particular care. In the long term, the large amount of sugar in the stronger bags can also damage the peritoneal membrane. For these reasons you will probably be advised to avoid using the stronger bags unless it is really necessary. It is easier to achieve this if you stick to your fluid allowance (see Chapter 7 for more information on fluid balance).

## ENERGY IN THE DIET

The energy we get from food is measured in kilocalories (usually referred to simply as 'calories'), and varies depending on the different nutrients that the food contains (see the box below). Be aware that alcohol also contains calories.

| | |
|---|---|
| Fat: | 9 (kilo) calories per gram |
| Carbohydrate (sugar and starches): | 4 (kilo) calories per gram |
| Protein: | 4 (kilo) calories per gram |
| Alcohol: | 7 (kilo) calories per gram |

*Energy from fat*

Fat is the most concentrated form of energy or calories. Weight for weight, it has over twice the energy of carbohydrates or protein. It is important to know this if you need to gain or lose weight. This is the theory behind low-fat diets; they cut out fat and use reduced-fat products to lower the total number of calories you eat.

If you are underweight, or have a poor appetite and are unable to eat large quantities of food, you may want your diet to be richer in energy. Eating more fatty foods, such as extra butter, margarine, oil or full-fat products such as full-cream milk instead of skimmed milk, can help. Other examples of fatty foods include cream, pastry and fried foods. If you are concerned about heart health, try to use more of the unsaturated fats and oils (such as sunflower, corn and olive oils and margarines) instead of saturated fats (such as ghee, butter, palm oil or lard).

*Energy from carbohydrates*

There are two types of carbohydrates, starches and sugars. As well as being a good source of energy, starchy foods can be naturally low in fat and

| *Some examples of starchy and sugary foods* | |
|---|---|
| **Starchy foods** | **Sugars/sugary foods** |
| Bread | Sucrose |
| Potato | Glucose |
| Rice | Fructose |
| Pasta | White sugar |
| Noodles | Brown sugar |
| Yam | Demerara sugar |
| Breakfast cereals (plain) | Honey |
| Plantain | Maltodextrins |
| Chapatti | Molasses |
| Polenta | Jam, jelly, marmalade |
| Couscous | Sweets (boiled, chews, mints, etc.) |
| Oats | Turkish delight |
| | Full sugar fizzy drinks and squash |

provide many essential nutrients such as B vitamins and some protein. Wholegrain varieties also provide fibre to prevent constipation and tend to be more filling. Most sugar, however, is found in processed foods such as sweets, cakes and fizzy drinks, which don't have many other nutrients.

Generally, the recommendation is to take most of your energy in the form of high-fibre, starchy foods such as wholemeal bread and pasta, brown rice and wholegrain cereals. It is also beneficial to eat less food that is high in added sugar, especially if you are trying to lose weight. Ways to reduce your sugar intake can be seen in the table below.

On the other hand, if you need to put on weight, it can be helpful to eat more sugary foods. This is because they tend to be high in calories and not very filling. You may also find that you can often manage a sweet dessert

| Foods high and low in sugar | |
| --- | --- |
| **Higher sugar choices** | **Lower sugar choices** |
| Standard squashes and fizzy drinks | Diet, low-calorie, 'sugar-free', 'no added sugar' drinks/squashes/fizzy drinks |
| Sucrose<br>Add sugar/jam/honey/syrup<br>to foods and drinks | Choose artificial sweeteners<br>e.g. Canderel/Hermesetas/Sweetex or<br>shop's own brand of saccharin-based<br>or aspartame-based sweetener for<br>desserts and drinks |
| Standard yoghurts<br>(Note: low-fat yoghurts may<br>still be high in sugar) | Diet or 'lite' yoghurts |
| Fruit tinned in syrup | Fruit tinned in fruit juice<br>(Note: these may need to be drained<br>if you are on a low-potassium diet) |
| Standard milk puddings<br>and desserts | Reduced sugar desserts |
| Sugar-coated or<br>cream-filled biscuits | Plain biscuits e.g. rich tea<br>or wholemeal biscuits |
| Sugar-coated breakfast cereals | Plain cereals e.g. Weetabix,<br>Shredded Wheat, cornflakes, porridge |

or pudding even though you can't finish your main course. You can use the table on the previous page to pick out foods which are high or low in sugar. If you have diabetes, you should check with your dietitian before including sugar or sugary foods in your diet.

### Energy from protein
Protein is needed to keep the body tissues healthy, as well as for growth and healing. If we don't eat enough energy from fats and carbohydrate, our bodies will use protein for energy, causing weight loss and muscle wasting. As a general rule, the aim is to eat enough calories from fat and carbohydrate to prevent protein from being used in this way.

### High energy supplements
Some people with kidney failure find it difficult to eat enough food to give them all the energy they need. There are special energy supplements available on prescription to help with this. They come in the form of powders (to mix with food and drinks) or as liquid supplements. Ask your doctor, nurse or dietitian if you think you need an energy supplement.

# 3
# Protein

## WHAT IS IT?

Protein is important for normal function, growth and repair of all parts of the body, including the skin, muscles, blood and internal organs. Milk, meat, fish, eggs and soya beans are all rich in protein. Many other foods, such as bread, pasta, beans, nuts, lentils and peas, contain protein in smaller amounts.

Proteins are made up of smaller units called amino acids. Different proteins contain different amino acids. Some of these can be made by the body but others, known as 'essential amino acids', cannot. This is why it is important to eat a variety of protein-containing foods to make sure that you get all of the amino acids you need.

## WHAT HAPPENS IN KIDNEY FAILURE?

When your kidneys fail, your body becomes less efficient at using the protein you eat. At the same time, it is not uncommon to lose your appetite, making it harder to eat enough protein. There may also be restrictions on what you can eat (such as having to eat less phosphate and potassium) that can make it even harder to eat enough protein, as many protein-rich foods also contain a large amount of these substances. These factors can cause loss of muscle from the body (muscle wasting) in many people with kidney failure.

## HOW MUCH PROTEIN SHOULD YOU EAT?

Most people with kidney failure who are not on dialysis need to eat a moderate amount of protein. In practice, this means including a portion of protein-rich food at two meals each day and avoiding high-protein snacks between meals. However, there are some people who need to eat more protein-rich foods, either because their appetite is poor, or because they have another medical condition that causes them to need extra protein.

Some kidney specialists think that following a low-protein diet will slow down the rate at which the kidneys fail. They also think that a low-protein diet will help to reduce the build up of some of the toxic waste products normally dealt with by the kidneys. Other experts do not agree. They are also concerned that a low-protein diet is too restrictive for most people to follow and may lead to malnutrition. If you would like to find out more about the advantages and disadvantages of restricting protein in your diet, talk to your doctor or a specialist kidney dietitian.

## PROTEIN ON HAEMODIALYSIS

When people start haemodialysis, they are usually advised to increase the protein they eat. This is because a small amount of protein is lost during each haemodialysis session. The extra protein is also needed to keep people healthy and able to fight infections.

## PROTEIN ON PERITONEAL DIALYSIS

With peritoneal dialysis, protein is lost in the waste fluid that is drained out during each exchange. Infections such as peritonitis can cause even more protein to be lost and at the same time reduce appetite so less protein may be eaten. This means that people having peritoneal dialysis need more protein in their diet, and should be given advice on eating protein-rich foods.

---

☑*TRUE OR* ☒*FALSE ?*

I need to eat meat to get enough protein in my diet

☒ **FALSE** Vegetarians can get all the protein they need by choosing a good variety of foods and eating a balanced diet

---

## PROTEIN IN THE DIET

*What sort of food is best to eat?*
Food that contains the most protein, with the full range of amino acids, tends to come from animals – for example, meat, chicken, fish, eggs, milk and cheese. Some vegetarian foods (such as Quorn and tofu) are also rich in protein. Beans, lentils, pulses, nuts and some starchy foods also contain

protein, but it is less concentrated and will be missing one or more essential amino acids. This means that vegetarians (and particularly vegans) have to take care to choose a range of protein-rich foods to make sure that they eat enough protein of the right kind.

> ### Examples of vegetarian/vegan meals containing a good combination of protein foods
> * a chickpea curry served with rice
> * baked beans on toast
> * wheat noodles with stir-fried tofu

Some protein-rich food contains large amounts of phosphate and potassium. If you need to follow a low-phosphate diet, you may need to limit certain high-protein foods (such as offal, shellfish along with dairy foods such as milk, hard cheese and eggs). On a low-potassium diet you may need to restrict milk, beans and lentils. This will vary, so ask your dietitian for advice for balancing your protein needs with any dietary restrictions. There is more information on potassium in Chapter 4 and on phosphate in Chapter 5.

### High protein supplements
Some people with kidney failure find it difficult to take enough protein in their diet. There are special food supplements available on prescription to help overcome this problem. These will usually be prescribed by your GP on the advice of the renal dietitian. Other protein supplements are widely available in health food shops, gyms and other outlets, but some may be harmful (see also page 52). You should check with your doctor or dietitian before taking any of these products.

# 4
# Potassium

## WHAT IS IT?

Potassium (the symbol 'K' is often used) is a mineral that is vital for life. The level in the body is normally controlled by the kidneys. This is important for the normal function of all nerves and muscles, including the heart. Potassium is present in a wide variety of foods including fruit, vegetables, meat and milk.

## WHAT HAPPENS IN KIDNEY FAILURE?

When kidneys fail, they can no longer control potassium levels. This can lead to a blood potassium level which is above or below the usual range of 3.5–5.0 mmol/litre. (Your hospital may use a slightly different normal range, so do check this locally.) High potassium levels (hyperkalaemia) can interfere with normal muscle and nerve function and cause the heart to beat irregularly. Low potassium levels (hypokalaemia) can also cause problems.

## DO YOU NEED A LOW-POTASSIUM DIET?

If your potassium level is normal, you won't need a low-potassium diet. If your potassium level is too high, it can be controlled by reducing the amount of potassium you eat. Your doctor may ask you to see a dietitian who will help you cut down on potassium without losing out on taste or other important nutrients.

## POTASSIUM ON HAEMODIALYSIS

Haemodialysis is very efficient at removing potassium, but is usually provided only three times each week. Because of this, many people need to follow a low-potassium diet in order to prevent potassium levels from building up between haemodialysis sessions. However, not everyone on haemodialysis will be on a low-potassium diet.

## POTASSIUM ON PERITONEAL DIALYSIS

Peritoneal dialysis works continuously, which usually prevents the blood potassium level from becoming too high. On the other hand, peritoneal dialysis will continue to remove potassium from the blood even if you don't eat much potassium, and this may cause blood levels to fall too low. So, if you are on peritoneal dialysis, you may not need to restrict your potassium intake. Do discuss this with your dietitian, especially if you are just starting this form of dialysis.

| *Recommended target values for blood potassium levels* (Renal Association: *Treatment of adults and children with chronic renal failure*, 3rd Edition, 2002) | |
| --- | --- |
| Pre-dialysis | 3.5–5.0 mmol/L (or local normal values) |
| Haemodialysis | 3.5–6.5 mmol/L (from a blood test immediately before a haemodialysis session) |
| Peritoneal dialysis | 3.5–5.5 mmol/L |
| **Note:** The level that is suitable for you as an individual may be slightly different. You should discuss your own levels with your doctor or dietitian. You can find out your blood potassium level by asking for the results of your blood tests. | |

## OTHER CAUSES OF ABNORMAL POTASSIUM LEVELS

A high potassium level may not always be caused by diet. Other factors include drugs such as ACE inhibitors (a type of blood pressure tablet), constipation, not getting enough dialysis, muscle breakdown, blood transfusions and poorly controlled diabetes. Low potassium levels can develop as a result of certain diuretics (water tablets) as well as a low dietary intake of potassium.

## CHOOSING A LOW-POTASSIUM DIET

*Which foods contain potassium?*
Most food contains potassium. Foods are often ranked as 'high', 'medium' or 'low', depending on the level of potassium in a typical serving.

However, you may find some variations in the advice given by different hospitals. Check with your own hospital's recommendations and discuss any queries with your dietitian.

If you need to eat less potassium, you will be advised to limit certain high-potassium foods or avoid them altogether. High potassium foods include coffee, chocolate, dried fruit and bananas. Some foods, such as milk and certain fruits and vegetables, contain a moderate level of potassium and provide other important nutrients. You will be given guidelines on the amounts and types of these foods that you can eat. There are also many foods that are low in potassium which can be eaten freely or as usual, such as tea, bread, rice, pasta and noodles.

Don't restrict your potassium intake unless you are advised to do so. Many high-potassium foods, such as fruit and vegetables, are an important part of a healthy diet.

### Are cooking methods important?
Potassium dissolves in water, so it is possible to reduce the amount in potatoes, yams and other vegetables by boiling them in plenty of water. Some of the potassium is lost into the water, which can then be thrown away. On the other hand, cooking methods such as steaming, microwaving, baking, roasting and frying use very little or no water and do not remove potassium. If you are on a low-potassium diet you will usually be asked to boil your vegetables and potatoes before eating, baking, roasting or adding to stews, curries, soups and the like.

### Food labelling
Potassium isn't usually listed on food labels, but you can check the ingredient list on the packet so that you can avoid items containing a lot of potassium. The ingredients are listed in order of the amount in the food. For example if a frozen vegetable curry lists spinach and potatoes (high-potassium vegetables) as the first two ingredients, it will be high in potassium so you might well choose not to eat it. Alternatively, you could compensate by serving the curry with a low-potassium side dish, such as rice or bread. You should avoid any foods labelled as containing salt substitutes such as LoSalt, Ruthmol, etc. These may be used in products advertising themselves as 'low in salt' or 'low in sodium, but they do contain a lot of potassium. (For more information on food labelling, see pages 64–8.)

*Choosing and adapting recipes*

The recipes in this book will help you to make the most of the vegetables, fruit and other foods that are lower in potassium and to give you plenty of ways to make them interesting and tasty. You should also find plenty of ideas to help you to adapt your own favourite dishes and recipes to make them lower in potassium.

*Summary Table*

Overleaf is a summary of some general guidelines for eating a restricted potassium diet based on the main food groups. Your dietitian or local hospital will be able to provide you with more information.

POTASSIUM CHECKLIST

| Group | Examples of food in this group | Message |
|---|---|---|
| **Starchy foods** | Bread, chapatti, couscous, pasta, rice, noodles, breakfast cereals, potatoes, yam, plantain | These are energy foods. They should make up the bulk of your diet. Include a portion at every meal |
| **Fruits and vegtables** | Fresh, frozen, canned and dried fruits and vegetables | Can be high in potassium but rich in vitamins, minerals and fibre. Generally limited but not avoided |
| **Milk and dairy produce** | Milk (whole/semi/ skimmed), ice cream, yoghurt, soya milk, cheese, margarine, butter, cream | An important source of protein and calcium. Contains a moderate level of potassium |
| **Protein foods** | Meat, poultry, fish, eggs, nuts, beans, lentils, tofu | Can be high in potassium but valuable sources of protein, vitamins and minerals, so many not restricted |
| **Snacks and and desserts** | Biscuits, cakes, sweets, chocolates, crisps, pakora | High in fat and/or sugar |
| **Drinks** | Alcohol, fruit juice, coffee, tea, malted drinks, fizzy drinks, fruit squash, hot chocolate | May need to be counted as part of a fluid allowance |
| **Other** | Jam, sauces, pickles, seasonings, gravy, Marmite, stock cubes, etc. | Provide flavour, but often of low nutritional value |

| *Foods to limit or avoid* | *Recommendations* |
|---|---|
| Restrict intake of starchy vegetables e.g. Potatoes, yam, plantain. Avoid cereals or breads containing dried fruit, nuts or chocolate | Boil starchy vegetables in large volume of water, and discard the water before eating or cooking further. FIll up on other starchy foods, e.g. bread, pasta, rice |
| Limit certain high-potassium sources, e.g. avocado, bananas, dried fruit, rhubarb, blackcurrants, spinach, parsnips, okra, tomato purée, Brussels sprouts | Boil vegetables in plenty of water and discard water. Avoid steaming, microwaving, baking. Parboil vegetables before stir-frying or adding to stews/curries. Limit tomatoes used in cooking |
| Limit milk intake; limit milky puddings and yoghurts. Avoid evaporated and condensed milk and milk powder | Keep to your daily allowances recommended by your dietitian |
| Avoid fish tinned in tomatoes. Avoid nuts | Dried/tinned beans and lentils are a useful protein source for vegetarians but avoid if meal contains meat, poultry or fish |
| Avoid potato- or gram-flour-based crisps and snacks. Avoid chocolate, fudge, liquorice. Avoid biscuits and cakes containing dried fruit, nuts, chocolate | Lower potassium snacks include plain, jam and cream biscuits and cakes, wheat- or maize-based snacks |
| Limit beer, cider, coffee and fruit juice. Avoid chocolate or malted drinks | Many drinks very low in potassium and can be taken normally |
| Avoid salt substitutes, Marmite, stock cubes. Avoid tomato, brown and Worcester sauces | Experiment with alternative flavourings for food e.g. dried and fresh herbs, spices, garlic, black pepper, vinegar |

POTASSIUM CHECKLIST

# 5
# Phosphate

## WHAT IS IT?

Phosphate (the symbol $PO_4$ is often used) is a form of the mineral phosphorous and is needed to help make, maintain and repair your bones. The kidneys normally control the amount of phosphate in the body. If you eat too much phosphate, you will get rid of it in your urine whereas, if you aren't eating enough, your kidneys will reduce the amount that you lose. In this way, the level of phosphate in your blood is regulated.

Phosphate is mainly found in protein-rich foods such as meat, fish, milk, cheese, eggs, yoghurt and nuts.

## WHAT HAPPENS IN KIDNEY FAILURE?

As kidney failure progresses, the kidneys lose their ability to control phosphate levels in the body. This can result in an increase in blood phosphate levels above the normal range of 0.8–1.4 mmol/litre (your hospital laboratory may use a slightly different normal range, so do check this locally).

High levels of phosphate in the blood can have two effects. Firstly, it may make you itch. Secondly, it stimulates the production of a hormone called parathyroid hormone (PTH). If too much PTH is produced, this will cause bone disease, bone pain and damaged blood vessels in the long term.

## DO YOU NEED A LOW-PHOSPHATE DIET?

When your kidneys fail, they are less able to control the level of phosphate in your body. This makes it necessary for you to limit the amount of phosphate you take in from food, both by being careful about what you eat and by taking phosphate-binding tablets. These tablets combine with the phosphate in the food and prevent it being absorbed into the blood. They are taken with meals and snacks containing phosphate.

Examples of phosphate binders include Calcichew (calcium carbonate), Phosex (calcium acetate) and Renagel (sevelamer). Your pharmacist, specialist kidney doctor or dietitian can advise you about taking phosphate binders.

Most people with mild to moderate kidney failure are able to control their blood phosphate levels and will not be advised to go on a special diet. However, some people may still benefit from eating less phosphate at this stage, especially if they tend to have a particularly high phosphate intake.

With more advanced kidney failure, phosphate levels in the blood may start to rise. At this point, most people need to reduce the amount of phosphate they eat. If you are in this position, the best thing to do is ask a dietitian for advice on reducing the overall phosphate content of your meals while ensuring that you continue to eat a balanced diet. You may also be asked to start taking phosphate-binding tablets with your food.

---

## ☑*TRUE OR* ☒*FALSE ?*

I do not need to take my phosphate binders with every meal.

☑ **TRUE** Depends on the food you are eating. You only need to take your binders with a meal or snack which contains a significant amount of phosphate. For example, you should take them with egg on toast, but not with jam on toast. (It is the egg, not the toast, that contains phosphate).

---

## PHOSPHATE ON DIALYSIS

Dialysis is not very good at removing phosphate from the blood. So most people on dialysis will need to eat less phosphate in order to control the level in their blood. This can be difficult as they usually need to eat plenty of protein and most high-protein foods are also high in phosphate. The challenge is to eat less phosphate, without reducing your intake of protein and other nutrients; helping you to achieve this is an important part of the dietitian's role. Most people on dialysis also take phosphate-binding tablets to help control phosphate levels.

### Low phosphate levels

Some people on dialysis have low phosphate levels (hypophos-phataemia). This can happen if you don't take in enough phosphate to balance the amount removed by dialysis. If you think your phosphate level is too low, see your doctor or dietitian to find out the cause and what to do about it.

## CHOOSING A LOW PHOSPHATE DIET

### Which foods contain phosphate?

High phosphate foods include meat, fish, eggs, nuts and dairy foods such as milk, cheese and yoghurt. These foods are also good sources of protein, calcium, vitamins and minerals as well as being tasty and widely used. This means many foods containing phosphate are not restricted on a low-phosphate diet. However, you may be asked to limit the amount of dairy foods and eggs you eat, as well as nuts, offal, shellfish, oily fish and fish with edible bones (e.g. whitebait, anchovies, tinned salmon). For more information see the table at the end of this chapter – but do check with your doctor or dietitian before starting a low-phosphate diet.

### Food labelling

You can't use food labels to check for phosphate content of food as it will not be listed. Instead check the ingredients in the food to see whether they are high in phosphate. You might want to limit or avoid dishes that contain a high-phosphate food, or make sure you compensate by eating reduced amounts of phosphate in other dishes or meals. For example, a frozen meal of macaroni cheese will contain some milk and hard cheese that need to be taken into account; alternatively you may decide to choose a pasta dish that doesn't contain any of those ingredients.

### Choosing and adapting recipes

White fish (e.g. cod, haddock, plaice), egg whites, cream, cream cheese and cottage cheese are low in phosphate. We have tried to include recipes in this book that will provide plenty of ideas for using these foods. You should find that you can use some of the ideas and tips given to reduce the phosphate content of your own favourite recipes. Some suggestions are listed in the box on the next page.

On pages 26–7, you will find a summary of general guidelines for eating a restricted phosphate diet based on the main food groups.

## Lowering the phosphate content of your food

- Halve the amount of cheddar cheese but use mature or strong cheddar for flavour

- Halve the amount of cheese in a cheese sauce and add some mustard to boost the flavour

- Use cream or crème fraîche with desserts instead of custard

- Substitute cream, cream cheese or crème fraîche for some of the milk when making milky sauces or desserts. This will increase the calorie and fat content of the dish, but there are also low-fat/low-calorie alternatives available

- Egg yolks contain more phosphate than the whites: experiment by missing out some (or all) of the egg yolks from dishes such as omelettes, scrambled egg, egg mayonnaise etc.

- If you find cottage cheese and cream cheese bland, try adding some flavourings (see our section on sandwiches for some ideas)

- Remove bones from tinned fish such as salmon and pilchards – don't mash them in with the flesh

**PHOSPHATE CHECKLIST**

| Group | Examples of food in this group | Message |
|---|---|---|
| Starchy foods | Bread, chapatti, pasta, rice, noodles, breakfast cereals, potatoes, yam, plantain | These are energy foods; they should make up the bulk of your diet. Include a portion at every meal |
| Fruits and vegtables | Fresh, frozen, canned and dried fruits and vegetables | Low in phosphate, rich in vitamins minerals and fibre. May be limited if you are on a potassium restriction |
| Milk and dairy produce | Milk (whole/semi/ skimmed), ice cream, yoghurt, soya milk, cheese, margarine, butter, cream | An important source of protein, calcium and other nutrients. Tend to be high in phosphate |
| Protein foods | Meat, poultry, fish, eggs, nuts, beans, lentils, tofu | Moderately high in phosphate but a good source of protein, minerals and other nutrients |
| Snacks and and desserts | Biscuits, cakes, sweets, chocolates, crisps, pakora | High in fat and/or sugar |
| Drinks | Alcohol, fruit juice, coffee, tea, malted drinks, fizzy drinks, fruit squash, hot chocolate | May need to be counted as part of a fluid allowance |
| Other | Includes jams, honey, sauces, pickles, herbs, spices, vinegar, fats, oils | Most unlimited unless conflicting with other dietary restrictions |

| Foods to limit or avoid | Recommendations |
|---|---|
| Avoid cereals or breads containing nuts or chocolate | |
| Limit milk intake. Limit milky puddings, cheese and yoghurts. Avoid processed cheese, evaporated and condensed milk and milk powder | Keep to your daily allowance as recommended by your dietitian. Cream, butter and margarines are low in phosphate. Cottage and cream cheese are lower in phosphate than other cheeses |
| Avoid nuts. Limit offal and processed meats. Limit oily fish and shellfish. Limit eggs | Beans and lentils are useful protein source for vegetarians but reduce or avoid if meal contains meat or fish |
| Limit nuts and gram-flour-based snacks. Limit chocolate, fudge. Limit biscuits and cakes containing nuts, toffee, chocolate | Lower phosphate snacks include plain, jam and cream biscuits and cakes |
| Avoid chocolate and malted drinks. Milky drinks counted within milk allowance | Many drinks very low in phosphate and can be taken normally |
| Limit chocolate spread. Avoid baking powder | |

PHOSPHATE CHECKLIST

# 6
# Salt (sodium)

## WHAT IS IT?

Salt is the name commonly used for 'sodium chloride', which is naturally found in some foods and is added to others to add flavour and preserve them. Sodium is a part of salt, and is important in our bodies for fluid balance and blood pressure control, as well as ensuring our muscles and nerves work properly.

## HOW MUCH SALT DO WE NEED?

Although salt is important for the body to function, we only need a very small amount. Currently in the UK, we eat an average of around 10 grams (the equivalent of two teaspoons) of salt every day. For good health it would be better to cut this to about 6 grams of salt each day.

## WHY REDUCE YOUR SALT INTAKE?

Eating less salt can prevent or treat high blood pressure (hypertension) which will protect against strokes, heart attacks and further damage to the kidneys. It is also thought to reduce the risk of developing stomach cancer and bone disease.

Cutting down on salt can also help to prevent fluid retention and to control thirst in people who need to restrict their fluid intake (see Chapter 7).

## HOW CAN YOU REDUCE THE AMOUNT OF SALT YOU EAT?

Reducing the amount of salt you eat may make food taste bland at first, but after about 6–8 weeks, your tastebuds will adjust to it. If you speak to other people who have cut down on salt, they often say that they now dislike the taste of salty foods and prefer foods made with less salt.

There are three main ways to reduce your salt intake:

- eat fewer processed foods and fewer foods that are naturally high in salt;
- do not add salt at the table;
- use less salt in cooking.

## EATING FEWER SALTY FOODS

Surprisingly most of the salt we eat is hidden in processed foods. This accounts for three quarters of our total intake. Only one quarter of the salt we eat comes from the salt that we add either at the table or in cooking.

Eating less of these types of food will help to cut down on salt in your diet. Fortunately, there is usually a lower salt food that you can try instead. (See the table on page 30.)

*Working out whether foods are high in salt?*
Many processed foods contain a high level of salt, so it is important to check food labels. At the moment most food labels state only the amount of sodium in the food. To compare the salt content of different foods, look for the 'sodium per 100 g' value on the label.

---

### ☑*TRUE OR* ☒*FALSE ?*

Food labelled as having 'no added salt' means it is low in salt.

☒ **FALSE** This term just means no salt has been added in the cooking process. It does not always mean that it is low in salt.
Other labelling terms are:
**Reduced sodium** Means it is at least 25 per cent lower in sodium than the standard product. The food could still be high in sodium, e.g. low-sodium soy sauce is lower in sodium than standard soy sauce, but it is still very salty
**Low in sodium** Means a sodium content of less than 0.04 g per 100 g of food. This is a 'genuinely' low-salt food

---

## Reducing your intake of salty foods

| Eat less | Choose instead |
|---|---|
| Processed and cured meats e.g. ham, bacon, sausages and tinned meats | Plain roast or grilled meat – cooked without added salt |
| Smoked fish | Unsmoked fresh or frozen fish; tinned fish (preferably tinned in spring water) |
| Ready made, tinned, packet or instant soups. Meat and vegetable extracts such as Marmite, Bovril and Oxo | Homemade soup with water, spices and herbs or other flavorings instead of stock cubes |
| Salted snacks such as crisps, salted peanuts, Bombay mix, chevra | Low-salt crackers, rice cakes or crisps, plain unsalted popcorn |
| Bottled sauces e.g. ketchup, salad cream, Worcester sauce, soya sauce | Try olive oil, vinegar or homemade French dressing. Low-sodium soya sauce is available and contains about one third less salt than the standard version |
| Cheese – including Cheddar, blue cheeses, Parmesan, Edam etc. | Cottage cheese, ricotta and cream cheese |
| Tinned vegetables in brine | Use fresh or frozen vegetables or those tinned in spring water |
| Pickles, stock cubes, salted flavourings | Use half the amount or avoid altogether, and use herbs and spices instead |

*What is 'a lot'? What is 'a little'?*
The salt content of foods can vary widely, as shown in the table below.

| Comparison of sodium contents in different foods | | | |
| --- | --- | --- | --- |
| **A LOT**<br>(More than 0.5 g sodium/100 g) | | **A LITTLE**<br>(Less than 0.1 g sodium/100 g) | |
| Food | Grams (g) sodium per 100 g food | Food | Grams (g) sodium per 100 g food |
| Salad cream | 1.1 | Vinegar | 0.02 |
| Cornflakes | 1.0 | Shredded Wheat | Less than 0.01 |
| Corned beef | 0.9 | Roast beef | 0.05 |
| Cream crackers | 0.6 | Matzo crackers | Less than 0.01 |
| Baked beans | 0.5 | Frozen green peas | Less than 0.01 |

## DO NOT ADD SALT AT THE TABLE

Try to get out of the habit of adding salt to food without tasting it. Watch for hidden salt in many sauces and condiments such as tomato ketchup, mustard, soy sauce, chutney, pickles and brown sauce. To help keep your salt intake down, try to use these sparingly or avoid them altogether.

You may have come across salt substitutes that are promoted as a healthy alternative to salt. Some of these such as 'Lo-Salt', 'Selora' or 'Ruthmol', are made with potassium, and are not suitable for patients on a low-potassium diet.

## REDUCE SALT IN COOKING

Try to cook with fresh food as often as possible rather than using ready-made or convenience foods or sauces. Remember that many manufactured flavourings can be high in salt, for example garlic or celery salt, sea salt, curry pastes and seasoning powders such as Cajun seasoning or tandoori powder.

You can experiment with herbs, spices and other flavourings to boost the taste of your food without relying on salt. Here are a few ideas for tasty combinations of flavourings with some familiar foods.

| *Using herbs and spices to flavour foods* | |
|---|---|
| **Roast meat** | Apple with pork; mustard or pepper with beef; tarragon with chicken; rosemary with lamb |
| **Grills** | Flavoured oil; lemon juice; garlic; honey; coriander |
| **Mince/stews** | Bouquet garni; bayleaf; basil; oregano; sage; cumin; garam masala |
| **Fish** | Parsley; dill; fresh coriander; vinegar; lemon or lime juice; turmeric; lemon grass |
| **Potatoes** | Mint; garlic; chopped chives; spring onions; bayleaf |
| **Vegetables** | Basil; oregano; chives; thyme; parsley |

# 7
# Fluid balance

## WHAT IS IT?

Healthy kidneys balance the level of fluid in your body. They remove excess fluid in the body in the form of urine. Most people know that if they drink several additional cups of tea or glasses of water they will find themselves passing more urine than usual. This urine will probably be very dilute or light in colour. Conversely, if you drink less than usual, or get very hot and sweaty, your body will become dry or dehydrated, your kidneys will produce less urine and it will be more concentrated or darker in colour.

## WHAT HAPPENS IN KIDNEY FAILURE?

As kidneys fail, they are no longer able to balance the level of fluid in the body. This leads to fluid retention. Too much fluid within the body can cause unpleasant side effects and lead to heart problems in the longer term. Too little fluid (dehydration) also causes problems such as low blood pressure and dizziness.

If you think that you have any of the symptoms of fluid overload (see the box below), you should report them to your medical team.

---

### Signs of fluid overload

Ankle swelling and oedema (water in the skin)

Shortness of breath (due to water around the lungs)

Raised blood pressure

Heart problems in the long term

Fluid-related weight gain

---

If you do need to restrict your intake, you will be told how much you can drink each day. The amount will vary between individuals, and may change over time (see the box below), so it is important to review your fluid allowance regularly with your kidney doctors and nurses.

---

### Factors affecting your fluid allowance

- The amount of urine you pass each day (this may change over time)
- Starting dialysis
- Type of dialysis
- Any period of illness
- Certain medications (especially diuretics or 'water tablets')

---

## FLUID BALANCE AND DIALYSIS

Dialysis removes any excess fluid from your body. Unfortunately dialysis is not as effective as healthy kidneys, and there is a limit to how much fluid can be removed. This means that most people on dialysis have to control the amount of fluid they take in, whether in the form of drinks or in certain foods.

Your kidney doctors and nurses will estimate how much extra fluid you have in your body. They can then work out your 'dry' weight. The 'dry' weight is the weight you would be if your kidneys were working normally and you had a normal level of fluid in your body. If you are retaining fluid, your body weight will increase in the same way as if you stepped on the scales carrying the extra fluid in a bucket. For example, 1 litre of extra fluid over your 'dry' weight will put your weight up by 1 kg; whereas 1 litre below will reduce it by 1 kg.

Sometimes it is hard to work out whether your weight is changing due to changes in the fluid in your body or whether it is due to changes in flesh weight (the amount of fat or muscle you have). If you experience a rapid increase in weight – say over 0.5 kg per day – this is likely to be due to fluid retention. Similarly, rapid weight loss is likely to be due to dehydration. Weight gain or loss due to changes in flesh weight tend to happen much more slowly. To help you and your healthcare team make these assessments, it is helpful to keep them informed of any significant changes to what you have been eating, or the amount of urine you have been passing.

## WHAT HAPPENS ON HAEMODIALYSIS?

If you are on haemodialysis, fluid is only removed during your dialysis sessions (usually three times a week). On the days between sessions, fluid builds up in your body. How much depends mainly on how much fluid you take in (as food or drink) during that time, and whether you are still passing any urine. You should try to limit the amount of fluid weight you gain between each dialysis session. As a general rule the amount of weight you can gain safely depends on your body size. In practice, this will usually represent a limit of anything between 1.5 kg to 3 kg above your dry weight (or less than 4% of your dry weight for those who are mathematically minded).

You will be given advice about your daily fluid allowance. This is the maximum amount of fluid you can take as drinks or in food.

*Q* I am on haemodialysis. How can I work out how much fluid I am allowed?

*A* If you are on haemodialysis, your daily fluid allowance is likely to be an amount equal to 500 ml plus an equivalent volume to the amount of urine you passed in the previous 24 hours. For example, if you pass 400 ml of urine per day, your total daily fluid allowance will be 400 ml + 500 ml, totaling 900 ml.

However, if you no longer pass urine, your daily fluid allowance will be 500 ml (approximately one pint) only.

## WHAT HAPPENS ON PERITONEAL DIALYSIS?

Unlike haemodialysis, peritoneal dialysis is continuous and fluid is being removed most of the time. However there is still a limit on how much fluid is removed each day, and on the amount of fluid you can take in. This is determined by each person's physical make-up and by the 'strength' or glucose concentration of each dialysis bag. The daily fluid allowance for people on peritoneal dialysis is usually about 800 mls plus the amount of urine passed in a 24-hour period. So for people who pass some urine (say around 1 litre/day) the daily fluid allowance would be 1800 mls, whereas for people who pass no urine at all, it would be 800 mls. People on peritoneal dialysis are usually advised to weigh themselves daily and to keep their weight within 1–2 kg of their 'dry' weight each day. If you are on this type of dialysis, you should ask your dialysis nurse or doctor to advise you what 'dry' weight you should be aiming for.

## YOUR FLUID ALLOWANCE

Many people find keeping within their fluid allowance is the hardest part of their renal diet. All cups and glasses vary in size. Measure the volume in the ones you use regularly to help you count your fluid intake, and see below for some standard sizes.

> ### *Handy fluid measures (1)*
>
> One teacup = 150 mls
> One hospital cup = 180 mls
> One small wine glass = 125 mls
> One mug = 250 mls
> Average can of fizzy drink = 330 mls
> One pint = 560 mls

Some people find it useful to get an idea of how much they would normally drink during the day. You can do this by keeping a measuring jug in your kitchen. Start each day with the jug empty. For every drink

> ### ☑ *TRUE OR* ☒ *FALSE ?*
>
> It is a bad idea to to eat rice or pasta as they absorb water.
>
> ☒ **FALSE** Almost all foods contain water! Rice and pasta are dried foods. When you cook them they simply reabsorb the water that was lost in the drying process. As they are both good sources of energy and naturally low in potassium and sodium, they are useful foods for people on dialysis so you are unlikely to need to restrict them.

you have, put the same quantity of water in the jug. You will then be able to see your total intake of fluid as the day goes on.

*What counts as fluid?*
All liquids in your diet need to be counted as part of your fluid allowance. These include tea, water, alcohol and milk on cereals. Your allowance also includes foods that contain a lot of fluid, such as gravy, soup, jelly, ice cream, stews and some dahls (see the box below).

---

### Handy fluid measures (2)

One tablespoon of gravy
or double cream = 15 mls
One ice cube = 20 mls
One scoop/brickette of ice cream = 50 mls
125 g portion of jelly or custard = 100 mls
Milk on cereals ( average) = 100 mls
One carton of yoghurt = 120 mls

---

*Tips to help with your fluid allowance*
In this book we have included recipes for a range of dishes that are low in salt and low in fluid to help you control your thirst and keep to your fluid allowance. Here are some practical tips that may help you keep to your fluid allowance. They have all been suggested by people on dialysis or by dietitians working with them.

---

### Tips to help you manage on a limited fluid intake

- Reduce your intake of salty and spicy foods as these foods will make you thirsty.
- Divide your fluid allowance evenly throughout the day.
- Use a smaller cup for drinks such as tea, squash etc. so that you can have a drink more frequently.
- Check which of your tablets may be taken with food to avoid using fluid to swallow them.

### Tips to help you manage on a limited fluid intake (cont'd)

- Try to drink when you are thirsty rather than out of habit. Get used to sipping your drinks, or use a straw to slow you down and prevent you gulping them too quickly.

- Avoid taking drinks with meals. Save them for between meals and for taking tablets.

- Use boiled/sherbet sweets, mints or chewing gum to freshen your mouth and stimulate production of saliva. If you have diabetes remember to choose the sugar-free varieties.

- Rinse your mouth with mouthwash or iced water, or clean your teeth to freshen your mouth.

- You may find sucking on ice cubes more satisfying than the same amount of water since it lasts longer. You can flavour ice cubes by making them out of squash or adding a drop of lemon juice.

- Try sucking on a slice of citrus fruits to quench your thirst.

- Eat fruit between or after meals to help moisten your mouth.

- When having tinned fruit, drain away the juice/ syrup (this will also reduce your potassium intake).

- Using plastic ice cubes can also be a way to reduce your fluid intake while still keeping your drinks chilled.

- If you drink to be sociable and feel you may drink a little more than you should, plan for this by drinking slightly less during that day and the following day.

- If you are choosing an alcoholic drink, remember spirits are lower in volume than beer or lager. However, if you are going to add a mixer (e.g. lemonade) this must also be counted in your allowance.

# 8
# Healthy living

## WHAT IS IT?

Healthy living involves a combination of healthy eating, keeping active and mobile, along with retaining a positive interest in life. Healthy eating means choosing a diet with the right balance of energy, nutrients and fibre to keep you as healthy as possible for as long as possible. Healthy living also involves keeping your weight at an appropriate level, following activities you enjoy and which keep you fit, as well as taking responsibility for your part in maintaining your own health.

## DO YOU NEED TO FOLLOW A HEALTHY DIET?

Most people with kidney failure will benefit from a healthy diet, for the following reasons:

❶ Some health problems will improve. For example, if your blood pressure is high, eating less salt and aiming for a healthy weight is an important part of your treatment plan. It will also help protect your kidneys from further damage.

❷ You can help to prevent and treat other conditions such as diabetes, high blood fats, high blood cholesterol level and obesity.

❸ You will make yourself fitter for dialysis or a transplant operation when the time for one of these arises.

## GENERAL TIPS FOR HEALTHY EATING

- **Eat regular meals including breakfast; don't skip meals**  This is good advice for everyone, whether you are overweight, underweight or about right. Pages 41–2 give information to help you work out your ideal weight. If you are underweight or have a small appetite, eating regularly and including extra snacks between meals is a very useful way to make sure you eat enough.

- **Eat less fat and fewer fatty foods** This will help to control cholesterol, which is important in reducing your risk of heart disease. If you are overweight then eating less fat can help you to lose weight.

- **If you eat fat, choose healthier fats** Eating unsaturated (polyunsaturated or monounsaturated) fats instead of saturated fats can lower your risk of heart disease by reducing your cholesterol level. Unsaturated fats usually come from plants, such as olive, rapeseed, sunflower or soya oils and margarines.

- **Eat oily fish regularly** The omega-3 oil found in oily fish can help to protect you against heart disease. Oily fish include herring, mackerel, salmon, sardines and trout; they are also a rich source of protein. If you are following a low-phosphate diet you may be asked eat less oily fish, but it should still be possible to include some in your diet.

- **Eat less sugar and fewer sugary foods** These foods tend to be high in energy (calories) and low in other nutrients, so should be avoided if you are overweight. However if you are underweight, feel nauseous or have a poor appetite they can be very useful. Sugary foods are often easy to eat and may tempt your appetite even when you have had enough of the main course. (You will know what we mean if you have ever felt completely full up after a large meal but still couldn't resist the dessert!) Also, sweet foods are often more appealing than savoury foods if you are suffering from taste changes. See Chapter 2 for more information and practical tips on sugar.

- **Eat foods rich in fibre** High fibre foods include wholegrain cereals, wholemeal bread and pasta, brown rice, pulses, lentils and fruit and vegetables. Eating fibre-rich food protects you against heart disease and cancer. It also helps to keep your bowels working normally and avoid constipation, which is particularly important if you are on peritoneal dialysis. However, some of these foods (in particular, some of the fruit and vegetables) are high in potassium. If you need to follow a low-potassium diet, ask your dietitian how you can include high-fibre foods safely in your diet.

- **Eat more fruit and vegetables** Fruit and vegetables are tasty, provide vitamins, minerals and fibre and can protect you against heart disease and cancer. However, they also contain potassium, in varying amounts. This means that if you have kidney disease or are on dialysis you should check with your doctor or dietitian before you increase your fruit and vegetable intake to make sure that your blood potassium levels will not be affected.

- **Eat less salt** We are all advised to eat less salt and this is true, too, for most people who have kidney failure. Anyone whose fluid allowance is restricted will find a low-salt diet helpful in controlling thirst. Avoid adding salt to food and in cooking, as well as keeping clear of salty foods such as processed meat, salted biscuits and bottled sauces. Chapter 6 includes plenty more information on cutting down on salt.

- **Drink alcohol in moderation** Unless your doctor advises you to avoid alcohol altogether, you should be able to include alcohol in moderate amounts if you wish. As a general guide, it is advisable to limit yourself to a maximum of 21 units per week for men (no more than 4 units in one day) and 14 units per week for women (no more than 3 units in one day). A unit is equal to half a pint of standard strength beer, a single pub measure of spirits or a standard glass of wine. Be aware that drinks you pour yourself are usually larger than standard pub measures. Some alcoholic drinks, such as cider and red wine, contain appreciable amounts of potassium. You may be advised to limit these if your blood potassium level is high. If you have been told to restrict your fluid intake, remember to include alcoholic drinks within your allowance.

## MAINTAINING A HEALTHY WEIGHT

A healthy weight is usually taken to mean the weight at which you have neither too much nor too little body fat. One way to estimate your healthy weight is to calculate your body mass index or BMI which compares your weight with your height (see the chart, overleaf). A BMI of between 20 and 25 is generally recommended as healthy so there will be a range of weights considered to be healthy for your particular height. A BMI of 26–30 is overweight, whereas a BMI over 30 indicates obesity.

$$\text{Body mass index} = \frac{\text{weight (kg)}}{\text{height (m)} \times \text{height (m)}}$$

Example: Fred is 1.66 m tall and weighs 78 kg

$$\text{BMI} = \frac{78}{1.66 \times 1.66} = 28$$

So Fred is overweight. A healthy weight range for this height would be 55–69 kg.

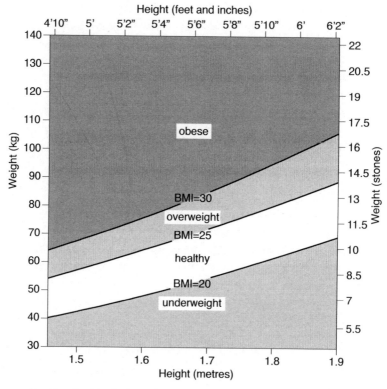

Use the chart or do the calculation above to find out your BMI.

Your BMI score:
below 20: underweight
20–25: ideal/healthy
25–30: overweight
30+: seriously overweight (obese)

## Weight changes in kidney disease

Weight loss and weight gain do not follow quite the same patterns if you have kidney failure. For example, you may retain water in your body which makes your ankles swell. The weight of this water will also mean that you appear to weigh more than you actually do. In this case, you will feel fat and 'swollen' but it is important not to 'diet' in the traditional sense; it is water rather than fat your body needs to lose. Indeed, if the swelling goes down, you may find you are much thinner than you thought. This is why people with kidney failure need to calculate their BMI using their 'dry weight' – the weight they would be without the extra fluid. Your doctor will be able to estimate how much water you are retaining and help you work out how much you should really weigh.

## Weight changes and dialysis

If you are on haemodialysis, you will find that your body regularly gains a few pounds or kilos between each dialysis session. This additional weight is fluid which needs to be removed during dialysis. Keeping to your fluid allowance will limit this fluid gain to safe levels. Gradual changes to your weight are more likely to be due to losses or gains of flesh weight.

If you are on peritoneal dialysis, you also need to be aware of the effect of fluid retention and changes to both flesh weight and overall weight. Some of the sugar in the dialysis bags used for peritoneal dialysis is absorbed by your body. The higher the strength of your dialysis bags, the more sugar you will absorb. This provides you with extra calories that can make you put on (flesh) weight. If you are concerned about this you should talk to your dialysis nurses. To limit the amount of sugar you absorb, you should make sure that you keep to your fluid allowance. This will help you avoid using strong bags unnecessarily.

---

### Case example 1: Mohammed

Mohammed has kidney disease and has gone off his food. However he is worried that he is overweight as none of his trousers fit, so has tried to cut down what he eats. When he goes to the clinic they explain that the weight he has gained is fluid which is making his legs and body swollen. They give him new tablets to get rid of the extra fluid. Now he notices that his legs look really thin so he must have been losing flesh weight while his appetite was poor.

---

*Case example 2: Mary*
When she arrives for haemodialysis Mary weighs 54 kg. Her dialysis nurse told her that she is too heavy as her dry weight is 51 kg. Then the dietitian told Mary to gain weight, as she should be 60 kg. Who is right?

*Answer:* both the nurse and the dietitian are right but they need to explain what they mean. The 3 kg weight that Mary has gained is fluid that needs to be removed by the haemodialysis machine. The dietitian thinks that Mary is too thin as her BMI is 17. She needs to gain (flesh) weight to give her a healthy BMI of at least 20. Therefore Mary needs to drink less and eat more.

*Case example 3: Donna*
Donna is on CAPD. She has recently given up smoking, generally feels really well and has a good appetite. She is finding that she is putting on weight so she has cut down even more on what she is drinking and has been told by her dialysis nurse that she is dehydrated. The dietitian explains that it is not water that is making her weight increase, but that she has become fatter because she is snacking more between meals.

   Donna goes back to following her previous fluid allowance, cuts back on her snacks and decides to start cycling with her son to get some exercise to help her lose the extra fat.

*Aim for a healthy weight*
If you are too fat and do need to lose weight, the best way to start is to follow the healthy eating guidelines (see pages 39–41). Make sure you are aiming for a realistic and healthy weight while increasing your activity levels as appropriate. If you feel too unwell to exercise it might be better to wait until you are feeling better before trying to lose weight. Some people find that group weight-loss classes or meetings are helpful but you will need to be careful that their dietary advice is in line with that from your doctor or dietitian. Remember, your dietitian will always be happy to discuss a suitable approach to weight loss with you and answer any questions you might have.

On the other hand, you may be underweight or have a small appetite and find yourself losing weight without meaning to. In this case you should try to see a dietitian to work out a treatment plan. You will probably be advised to eat more regularly, include snacks between meals and eat more high-energy (calorie) foods.

### Weight control and fad diets

> *'I've found a great diet to help me lose weight – should I use it?'*

Fad diets can be very tempting. They usually offer 'quick and easy' ways to lose weight, but weight loss should not be quick. Unfortunately, there is no magic solution to losing weight. If any product sounds too good to be true, it probably is – and it's just the same with weight-loss diets.

If you thinking about trying a weight-loss diet, you need to be careful – particularly if you have kidney failure. If any of the following points apply to the diet you are considering, then don't use it:

- Does it offer a 'miracle' cure or quick fix?

- Does it promote a limited number of particular foods such as cabbage, pineapple, grapefruit etc?

- Does it encourage you to eat an unbalanced diet which does not follow healthy eating guidelines, such as the high-protein, low-carbohydrate diets?

- Would it cost you a lot of money?

- Are there particular tablets, drinks or medication that you have to buy and which are only available from the individual or company promoting the diet?

'Quick fixes' rarely work, and if someone has additional health problems such as kidney failure they may cause real damage. You need to aim for permanent changes to both your diet and your weight. If you don't, you will find yourself gaining back the weight you have lost.

## EXERCISE AND ACTIVITY

We realise that exercise is not part of your diet, but it is difficult to talk about your diet without considering activity. Whether you are underweight, overweight or somewhere in between, it is important for you to think about the type and amount of exercise you do.

Exercise will help you build and maintain muscle. If you are overweight, being more active will help you to lose fat, gain muscle and reach and maintain a healthy weight.

Exercise can also help if you have trouble sleeping, feel anxious or depressed, and can lead to increased self-confidence, independence and a feeling of well-being. Exercise can improve bone strength, protect against osteoporosis and help with other conditions common in people with kidney disease, including anaemia, diabetes and high cholesterol. In fact, if you are not doing any form of exercise, you are missing out on a great benefit. It is cheap, easily available, and can prevent and treat many of the conditions from which you may suffer, now or in the future.

### What can you do?

Anything that makes you more active will provide you with exercise. Some ideas that involve you increasing your activity are:

- getting up to change channels on the TV instead of using the remote control;
- walking to the shops instead of driving;
- getting off the bus one or two stops earlier and walking the rest of the way;
- doing some housework;
- using the stairs instead of a lift or escalator;
- walking in the park, the countryside or even just around the block;
- performing 'chair exercises' (exercising while seated);
- asking the renal unit whether they have a pedal machine to attach to the bottom of the dialysis station, so you can 'pedal exercise' while you are having your dialysis session.

You could also take up an active pastime or learn a new skill. Lots of people with kidney failure enjoy a wide range of activities, whether or not they are on dialysis. Real-life examples include cycling, ballroom dancing, line dancing, golf, bowls, wheelchair basketball, wheelchair archery, aerobics, swimming, aqua-aerobics, clubbing, gardening, running and working out at the gym. Why not visit your local leisure centre, or ask staff and other patients at your Renal Unit for more ideas and advice on activities you might enjoy.

To become more active you will need to decide what you would like to do and make a real commitment to doing it. Whatever you choose to do, make sure it is something you enjoy. Start off gently and build up gradually – your aim is to try to make your body work a little harder, perhaps from a brisk walk rather than a stroll. As a general rule you shouldn't do anything that makes you too out of breath to talk and – obviously – you should avoid doing anything that hurts. Although you shouldn't worry if you haven't done any exercise for a long time, it is always a good idea to check with your GP or clinic doctor before starting any new form of exercise. Your doctor will also be able to advise you about suitable ways to increase your activity levels and direct you to information on local facilities.

# 9
# Vitamins, minerals and supplements

There are national government guidelines for vitamin, mineral and trace element requirements in health. However, very little is known about requirements in people who have kidney failure or are on dialysis. Some kidney doctors and dietitians prescribe multivitamins for the majority of their patients on dialysis. Others believe that vitamin supplements should be reserved for those people who have particular needs. You should discuss what is right for you with your doctor and dietitian. If your appetite is poor you may feel that you should have a vitamin supplement. However, you may also need advice on eating enough energy, protein and other nutrients rather than simply focusing on supplementing one or more vitamin or mineral.

If you take any vitamin or mineral supplements, herbal remedies or anything else that your doctor hasn't told you to take, it is important to let your doctor, renal pharmacist and dietitian know when you see them. Some can cause unpleasant side effects for people with kidney failure or other medical conditions. They may react badly when taken with your other medications, and either make you feel ill or prevent them working. Or they may contain substances that only healthy kidneys can cope with properly.

## VITAMINS

Vitamins are essential for health, and your body needs them in order to function properly. Eating a balanced diet (see pages 39–41) will help you get enough vitamins from your diet without the need for additional supplements.

There are two main categories of vitamins, those that are water-soluble (see table opposite) and those that are fat-soluble (see table on page 50).

## Water-soluble vitamins

| Name | Function | Dietary sources |
|---|---|---|
| B1 | Needed to convert food into energy | Breakfast cereals, bread, meat dairy produce, vegetables |
| B2 | Needed for growth and healthy body tissues, skin, eyes and nervous system | Milk, dairy produce, meat and cereals |
| Niacin | Needed to convert food into energy | Meat, dairy produce, breakfast cereals, bread, vegetables |
| B6 | Helps the body to make use of protein | Cereal, meat, potatoes, milk and dairy produce |
| Folic acid | Helps the body to make use of protein and build healthy cells | Cereals, vegetables, meat, milk and dairy produce |
| B12 | Needed for healthy blood cells and nerves | Meat, dairy produce, breakfast cereals, fish, eggs |
| C | Antioxidant, helps to protect cells and aids wound healing | Vegetables, potatoes, fruit, fruit juices |

Some water-soluble vitamins may be lost during dialysis, but supplements will not necessarily be needed as the losses are sometimes balanced out by reduced losses in the urine.

Among the fat-soluble vitamins, vitamin A supplements are unlikely to be needed as this vitamin is retained in the body by people who have kidney failure.

Vitamin D is particularly important as it cannot be made or used properly by the body unless you have healthy kidneys. A special vitamin D supplement (e.g. 1-alpha calcidol), which contains the active form of vitamin D, is often prescribed.

| Fat-soluble vitamins | | |
|---|---|---|
| **Name** | **Function** | **Dietary sources** |
| A | For cell development and healthy skin and eyes | Meat, offal, dairy produce, spreading fats, fish oils |
| D | Controlling calcium balance and bone development | Margarines and fat spreads, cereals, oily fish (in health, also made by the action of sunlight on skin) |
| E | Anti-oxidant, protects cells | Spreading fats, meat, fish, eggs, vegetable oils |
| K | Helps with blood clotting | Green leafy vegetables |

## MINERALS

Minerals are an essential part of a balanced diet. They can be divided into two groups: minerals we require in relatively large quantities and others, known as trace elements, which are needed in only very small amounts. Deficiencies of trace elements are unusual. However, they may occur on rare occasions if the diet is poor or very limited for a long period of time. See the tables on pages 51 and 52 for a summary of some minerals and trace elements.

Many of the minerals, including sodium, potassium, phosphorous and calcium, are removed through the kidneys. When the kidneys fail the body loses the ability to remove these minerals, which can build up and cause problems (see Chapters 4, 5 and 6).

### Iron

Iron helps to make red blood cells, which carry oxygen around the body. A reduced level of red blood cells below the normal level is known as anaemia. In healthy people, anaemia can be caused by not eating enough food containing iron, and is often treated by taking more iron in the diet, or with iron supplements. Anaemia is common in people with kidney failure, but this is mainly because of low levels of a substance called erythropoietin. Erythropoietin is produced by healthy kidneys and normally helps to make red blood cells. If extra iron is needed, this is given

## Minerals

| Name/Symbol | Function | Dietary sources |
| --- | --- | --- |
| Sodium (Na) | Essential part of the blood and other body fluids | Table salt, convenience foods, ready meals, fast food |
| Potassium (K) | Needed for normal muscle and nerve function | Meat, vegetables, fruit, potatoes |
| Iron (Fe) | Needed to make red blood cells | Red meat, dark green leafy vegetables |
| Calcium (Ca) | Essential for healthy teeth and bones | Dairy, cheese, milk, yoghurt |
| Phosphorus (P) | Needed for bones and energy production | Dairy, cheese, milk, yoghurt, offal shellfish |

as iron tablets or via a drip directly into the blood vessels. It is rare for anaemia in kidney failure to be caused by a diet low in iron, so make sure you eat a well balanced diet rather than focusing on eating any particular iron-rich foods.

*Calcium*
This mineral is important for the development of bones and teeth. If you are in good health, vitamin D will help your body use the calcium you eat. If you have kidney failure, however, low levels of vitamin D mean your body will find it difficult to absorb and use calcium. This may result in low blood calcium levels. If you are not eating enough, you may be given calcium supplements because it is difficult to increase calcium in the diet without taking in too much phosphate. For example, milk is a good source of calcium but is also high in phosphate and potassium. Some calcium may also be absorbed from calcium-containing phosphate binders.

Sodium, potassium and phosphorous are also minerals. See the relevant chapters for more information.

| *Trace elements* | | |
|---|---|---|
| Name/Symbol | Function | Dietary sources |
| Zinc (Zn) | Bone health, reproduction and digestion | Meat and pulses |
| Selenium (Se) | Functions as an antioxidant, protects cells | Meat fish and cereal grains |
| Chromium (Cr) | Helps with insulin activity and energy production | Meat, wholegrains, nuts and pulses |
| Manganese (Mn) | For healthy bones and other functions | Vegetables and tea |

## SUPPLEMENTS AND 'ALTERNATIVE' MEDICINES

A vast range of 'natural' or 'alternative' tablets, liquids and foods are now available from supermarkets, pharmacies and health food shops. If you do not have kidney failure, many of these will be safe and may even do you some good. But be warned: very little is known about how such medicines and other substances behave in your body, especially if your kidneys are not working properly. Some Chinese herbal medicines, for example, can be poisonous to the kidneys. They can make your kidney failure worse, and result in your needing dialysis sooner. So it is very important that you are careful about using any products like this, and if you are thinking about starting one make sure you discuss it with your kidney doctor or nurse first.

Do remember too that most of these products have only passed through simple food regulations, rather than the proper scientific testing required for all the medicines you might be prescribed.

# 10
# Different tastes

Being told that you have kidney failure doesn't have to mean your life won't be fun any more. This chapter gives advice to help you continue to enjoy going out and socialising, eating food you like, exploring different tastes and sharing in special occasions. By taking a few sensible precautions, you can continue to enjoy your chosen lifestyle to a much greater degree than you may have feared.

## EATING OUT

The two concerns which people with kidney failure usually find the most challenging when eating out are controlling their potassium levels and their fluid intake. This is because even short term rises in potassium levels, as well as in the amount of fluid in the body can be harmful. If you are trying to drink less, you will probably need to avoid salty foods too as these will tend to make you very thirsty. This doesn't mean that you can't treat yourself; just do so in moderation rather than going out for a big binge!

You may find that you can be more relaxed about other restrictions, including phosphate. Just how relaxed will really depend on how often you eat out. An occasional meal is unlikely to make much difference to your overall diet. But if you eat out at least once a week, you may need to choose your menu with a bit more care. Just as at home, your choices will depend on your own particular tastes, medical condition, blood results and lifestyle.

For many people, a special meal is just not special without a drink or two so try to plan for this if you can (see tips overleaf). Remember too that it is not just drinks (alcoholic or otherwise) that contain fluid. Include any soups, sauces, gravy, custard and other 'liquid' foods within your fluid allowance. Some drinks, such as fruit juices, coffee, beer, red wine and cider, are also high in potassium. If you are watching your potassium intake try fizzy drinks, bottled waters, tea, white wine and spirits instead.

***Tip:*** Try to reduce the amount you drink during 24 hours before a meal out or party where you may want to drink more than usual. You may also like to try this if you know that you will be eating a salty meal (pepperoni pizza or sausages, for example). This way, you will be able to have an extra drink after eating.

---

### ALCOHOL: SOME TIPS

- Check with your doctor or renal pharmacist that it is safe for you to drink alcohol with the medications you are on

- 'Shorts' are generally low in potassium, as well as in volume. But if you add a mixer, such as tonic water, don't forget to include this in your allowance

- Beer and wine are generally higher in both potassium and fluid, so you will need to think about what else you can cut down on to make up for this in your overall intake

---

### Asking ahead

Preparing yourself, and the people who are cooking for you, can make all the difference. For example:

- If you are going to a restaurant, try to contact the manager in advance. Ask about the choice of food, and discuss any special arrangements that might be needed.

- If you have been invited to someone else's home, you will make meal planning much easier for your hosts if you phone ahead to discuss what you can and can't eat.

- If you know that you might be eating a less suitable food for dinner at a friend's house you might just decide that you will be more careful during the day to compensate. For example, if you are on a low-potassium diet you might avoid eating fruit at lunchtime if you are having mushrooms or another high-potassium vegetable later that evening.

- A few simple changes to the way food is prepared and served can make a meal much easier for you to eat. Butter, sauces, gravy and salad dressings can be served separately or left out altogether; a high-potassium vegetable or fruit may be changed for a low-potassium alternative; garnishes can be omitted.

## Do's and don't's for eating out

**DO** try to plan ahead – you may be able to adjust your diet before or after the meal out to allow for any foods and drinks that you would not normally have

**DO** consider how often you eat out when deciding how flexible to be with your diet

**DO** try to choose suitable foods when you are out. If you run into difficulties concentrate on avoiding excess potassium, fluid and salt (if these restrictions apply to you)

**DO** remember to allow for alcoholic or non-alcoholic drinks as part of any social occasion or a meal out, especially if you are on a low-potassium or fluid-restricted diet

**DO** ask your host or waiter to serve the food appropriately. For example many sauces, dressings, garnishes and other extras can often be served separately or left out altogether

**DON'T** be afraid to ask the restaurant, café or takeaway to change a dish to suit your requirements. It's often worth telephoning ahead to check that they will have something that you are happy to eat

**DON'T** forget to ask your dietitian for advice on eating meals out and at special occasions. Dietitians will be happy to provide information (both for you and for your relatives and friends) that is geared to your own particular diet and needs

## FOODS FROM AROUND THE WORLD

Our multicultural society offers a wealth of eating experiences both at home and when eating out. Talking to your dietitian about the sort of diet you and your family like to eat can be very helpful. Don't worry about your dietitian being unfamiliar with a specific style of food, as he or she is likely to be keen to learn from you. You may well find you are soon working together, ensuring that any dietary changes don't have to stop you from eating your traditional or preferred foods.

Here are a few general tips to consider when choosing some of your favourite meals.

### Chinese and Thai

- Food from China and the Far East can be very salty. Avoid adding salt or salty sauces such as soy sauce or fish sauce. Ask for food without added MSG (monosodium glutamate), which is very high in salt.

- Plain boiled or steamed rice or noodles are suitable accompaniments to any meal, especially if you are on a low-potassium diet. Fried noodles and rice are higher in fat and energy so are best cooked in a 'healthy oil' such as sunflower, soya or rapeseed oils (see Chapter 8).

- If you need to restrict phosphate or potassium, avoid dishes containing peanuts, cashews and other nuts or ask the chef to leave them out when cooking your meal.

- Many typical flavourings (ginger, garlic, allspice, lemongrass) can be enjoyed freely for a delicious taste, particularly if you are on a low-salt diet.

- If you choose a dish such as a Thai curry which comes with plenty of sauce, try to leave most of the sauce behind in the serving dish. This will cut down on the amount of salt, fluid, fat and potassium that you eat.

- Stir fries may still be possible even on a low-potassium diet, especially if served with noodles or rice.

*Italian and Mediterranean*

- Pasta is low in potassium, phosphate and fat – which makes it a good choice – but you need to check the ingredients in the sauce. For example, a creamy sauce will raise the fat and calorie content while a tomato, mushroom or spinach-based sauce may be lower in fat but higher in potassium.

- Olive oil is a great choice if you are concerned about your risk of heart disease. It is a monounsaturated fat and an essential part of the 'Mediterranean diet', thought to be a particularly healthy style of eating. However, it is just as high in calories as any other fat.

- A low-salt dressing for fish, meat and vegetables can be made from balsamic vinegar or lemon juice, olive oil and black pepper. You can limit the oil or leave it out altogether if you are trying to lose weight.

- Bread is a great food and Italy and other Mediterranean countries have a wide range of breads to choose from. Try ciabatta, garlic bread, pitta bread or breadsticks as an accompaniment or starter. However, certain breads, such as foccacia and those with added ingredients such as olives, can be more salty than others.

- Avoid adding extra parmesan or other hard cheeses to dishes, wherever possible. Hard cheese is high in salt, phosphate and saturated fat and you may not even notice it has been left out. Soft cheeses such as ricotta, mascarpone and mozzarella are better choices, and you may be able to find low-fat versions to use at home.

- Pizza is another favourite. There is usually a wide range of toppings on offer so try to choose those which fit in best with your diet. For example, if a low-potassium diet has been recommended, you might want to avoid spinach or fresh mushrooms but have tinned mushrooms or pineapple instead. Additional salty ingredients such as anchovies are best avoided – as is extra cheese, either as a topping or in the 'stuffed-crust' or similar American-style pizzas.

## Indian/Indian subcontinent

- If your fluid allowance is restricted, try to choose the drier dishes with less sauce, such as bhuna, tandoori or biriyani style dishes. Also try keeping to the 'mild' or 'medium' dishes. The hotter the dish the more you will want to drink! If you choose to eat dishes with more liquid, try serving them with a slotted spoon to drain some away. This can also reduce the salt, fat and potassium content of the meal.

- Rice and chapattis or other plain breads such as plain naans, parathas and popodums are a good accompaniment to your meal. They are low in potassium, although their fat (and calorie) contents vary.

- If you make your pilau rice, chapattis or other breads at home, try to use the minimum amount of ghee or oil to keep the fat content down. However, if you need to put on weight, you may be advised to increase the amount of unsaturated oils (e.g. corn, sunflower or rapeseed oils) you use.

- There is a great choice of vegetables to sample. If you are on a potassium restriction try to keep within your vegetable allowance. Preboil vegetables if possible and limit the high-potassium vegetables, such as spinach, okra (ladies' fingers) and potato.

- If you are on a low-potassium or low-phosphate diet, limit nuts, including coconut and cashews, and gram (chickpea) flour based snacks such as pakora and Bombay mix.

## African/ Caribbean

- Stews and 'soups' are a traditional way to serve meat or fish with vegetables in one dish. Using a slotted spoon to dish up a portion of stew allows the liquid to drain away and reduces the fluid, salt and potassium content of the meal.

- If you are on a low-potassium diet, try to boil vegetables, potatoes and other starchy staples such as yams, sweet potato or plantain, before eating or adding them to stews and similar dishes.

- Other staples, such as plain rotis, rice, ground rice and couscous are low in potassium and fat.

- To cut down on your sodium (salt) intake, try to avoid dishes containing salted meats and fish. Fresh meat and fish are good alternatives. If you are preparing salted meat or fish at home, soak and rinse thoroughly in plenty of water to wash away some of the salt.

- A wide range of flavourings can be enjoyed including fresh and dried thyme, coriander and other herbs, garlic, chilli, allspice and other spices.

- If you are on a low-phosphate diet, limit the amount of shellfish you eat – preferably avoiding dried shrimp and prawns. Nuts, including coconut and peanuts, are usually limited if you are on a low-phosphate or low-potassium diet.

## CELEBRATIONS AND SPECIAL OCCASIONS

Family, national and religious holidays and celebrations can have a great influence on how we eat. From birthdays to bank holidays, Christmas to Chanukah, Eid to Diwali, many of these occasions have special foods and meals associated with them. Christmas, in particular, is associated with a vast range of seasonal foods that are available for several weeks of the year and will probably influence your diet whether or not Christmas is part of your own family traditions.

*Hints and tips for seasonal celebrations*

- Many special occasion foods tend to be high in potassium, especially around Christmas time. If you are on a potassium restriction, eat them sparingly to keep your potassium levels under control.

- Remember that all fluids count towards your fluid allowance, including alcohol, soup, gravy, custard and other sauces. Try to plan ahead to allow yourself a treat or two on the day.

- Roast meats such as turkey, pork, beef or lamb are a good choice eaten hot or cold. Try cooking with lemon, garlic, black pepper, spices or fresh herbs such as rosemary to add flavour instead of salt. Cranberry sauce, mint sauce and mustard can make good alternatives to gravy if you are watching your fluid intake.

- Potatoes, yam, plantain, sweet potatoes and parsnips are high in potassium and need to be boiled before eating or cooking further.

Keep portions small if there are a lot of other tempting high-potassium foods around, and help yourself to the lower potassium alternatives such as rice, pasta, couscous, noodles and breads.

- If you are on a potassium restriction try to limit the high-potassium vegetables you eat – including Brussels sprouts, spinach, mushrooms, callaloo and okra. Alternatives include cauliflower, broccoli, carrots, green peas and aubergine.

- If you can't resist fruit cake, mince pies, chocolate biscuits and cakes, nutty pastries, barfi or other high-potassium or high-phosphate desserts, keep to a small portion for that one-off treat. Trifle, cream cakes, meringues, jam tarts and shortbread are lower in phosphate and potassium but should still satisfy your sweet tooth!

- Most savoury nibbles are high in salt and will make those of you on a fluid restriction very thirsty. Crisps, pakora, nuts and Bombay mix are also high in potassium and phosphate. Lower potassium/phosphate nibbles include wheat-based snacks (e.g. tortilla chips, breadsticks and crackers). Avoid spicy flavours if they make you drink too much.

- Nuts, including peanuts and coconut, tend to be high in potassium and phosphate. Walnuts, pecans and chestnuts are a better choice but you should still have a few only.

- Dried fruit (figs, currants, dates, prunes etc.) are high in potassium but are a high-fibre, low-fat sweet treat if you do not need to restrict your potassium intake. Other special occasion fruit – such as pineapple, strawberries, satsumas and grapes – can make healthy sweet desserts and snacks. They can also help to counteract a dry mouth after too much salt. Tinned fruit (drained) is usually lower in potassium than fresh fruit.

# 11
# Practical hints

We've talked about the theory of eating with kidney failure; now it's time to turn it all into practice. This section of the book gives you some basic checklists: conversion charts, hints on using herbs and spices, advice on labelling and tips on food hygiene.

## CONVERSION CHARTS

All the conversions below are approximate. In all our recipes, spoon measurements are level unless otherwise stated.

| Weights | | Volume | |
|---|---|---|---|
| *Metric* | *Imperial* | *Metric* | *Imperial* |
| 7 g | ¼ oz | 5 ml | 1 teaspoon |
| 15 g | ½ oz | 15 ml | 1 tablespoon |
| 20 g | ¾ oz | 30 ml | 2 tablespoons |
| 25 g | 1 oz | 100 ml | 3½ fl oz |
| 40 g | 1½ oz | 125 ml | 4 fl oz |
| 50 g | 2 oz | 150 ml | ¼ pint |
| 75 g | 3 oz | 175 ml | 6 fl oz |
| 125 g | 4 oz | 200 ml | 7 fl oz |
| 150 g | 5 oz | 225 ml | 8 fl oz |
| 175 g | 6 oz | 250 ml | 9 fl oz |
| 200 g | 7 oz | 300 ml | ½ pint |
| 250 g | 8 oz | 350 ml | 12 fl oz |
| 275 g | 9 oz | 400 ml | 14 fl oz |
| 300 g | 10 oz | 450 ml | ¾ pint |
| 325 g | 11 oz | 500 ml | 18 fl oz |
| 375 g | 12 oz | 600 ml | 1 pint |
| 400 g | 13 oz | 700 ml | 1¼ pints |
| 425 g | 14 oz | 900 ml | 1½ pints |
| 450 g | 15 oz | 1 litre | 1¾ pints |
| 500 g | 17½ oz | 2 litres | 3½ pints |
| 1 kg | 2 lb 3 oz | 2.75 litres | 5 pints |

## Measurements

| Metric | Imperial |
|--------|----------|
| 5 mm | ¼ inch |
| 1 cm | ½ inch |
| 2 cm | 1 inch |
| 5 cm | 2 inches |
| 7 cm | 3 inches |
| 10 cm | 4 inches |
| 12 cm | 5 inches |
| 15 cm | 6 inches |
| 18 cm | 7 inches |
| 20 cm | 8 inches |
| 23 cm | 9 inches |
| 25 cm | 10 inches |
| 28 cm | 11 inches |
| 30 cm | 12 inches |

## Oven temperatures

(For fan ovens, adjust the cooking temperature in accordance with the manufacturer's instructions)

| Celsius | Fahrenheit | Gas Mark | Description |
|---------|-----------|----------|-------------|
| 110°C | 225°F | ¼ | cool |
| 120°C | 250°F | ½ | cool |
| 140°C | 275°F | 1 | very low |
| 150°C | 300°F | 2 | very low |
| 160°C | 325°F | 3 | low |
| 180°C | 350°F | 4 | moderate |
| 190°C | 375°F | 5 | moderate |
| 200°C | 400°F | 6 | mod hot |
| 220°C | 425°F | 7 | hot |
| 230°C | 450°F | 8 | hot |
| 240°C | 475°F | 9 | very hot |

## FLAVOURING WITH HERBS AND SPICES

You can use herbs and spices to help to reduce your salt intake without losing out on flavour. In our recipes we have tried to cut out or minimise the addition of salt as far as possible. Below is a list of some other suggestions you may also wish to try. As a rule of thumb, dried herbs and spices are best added into 'moist' foods such as soups, stews and sauces during cooking. Fresh herbs are widely available and add flavour to almost any dish. Some of the more delicate varieties such as coriander and basil are best added just before serving. Others, such as rosemary and thyme, release their flavour during cooking.

Many herbs are easy to grow, in the garden or on a window sill, and plants or seeds are readily available. Frozen herbs can be bought or made easily at home. Chop up the herbs and cover with a little water in an ice cube tray, then freeze. They will then be in convenient portion sizes for later use.

| Herbs | |
|---|---|
| Basil | **Fresh** – Add a chopped leaf or two to salad, or to pasta, stews and other hot dishes before serving; **Dried** – Add a pinch into stews or sprinkled on beef before roasting |
| Bay leaf | Use a couple of dried leaves in stocks and stews or when boiling potatoes |
| Chives | Chop a few fresh chives and add to a potato salad, cottage cheese, or serve with chicken or fish |
| Mint | Use a fresh sprig with vegetables or on a little lamb before grilling |
| Parsley | More than just a garnish … great with chicken, fish and vegetables |
| Sage | Add fresh or dried sage to home-made stuffings for pork or poultry; also good with roast vegetables or potatoes |
| Tarragon | A little fresh or dried tarragon goes well with chicken or fish; fresh tarragon is also tasty on a salad |
| Thyme | Use in stews, or in home-made stuffing for poultry and game |
| Mixed herbs | Try a pinch of dry or fresh, for stuffings, stews, omelettes, pizza |

| Spices | |
| --- | --- |
| **Cayenne** | A pinch in curry, or sprinkle a little on vegetables for a little 'zing' |
| **Cinnamon** | A sprinkling of ground cinnamon works well with stewed fruits or a pinch in your baking; or try mixed in plain yoghurt for a sweet taste without the sugar |
| **Ginger** | Sprinkle a little ground ginger on lamb or pork before grilling or roasting. Try ground or fresh ginger in curries, stir-fries and stewed fruit |
| **Mustard** | Rub mustard powder into beef before roasting for extra bite; add to cheese sauce, white sauce, other sauces and stews |
| **Paprika** | A fine dusting is an excellent garnish for chicken, white fish or rice |
| **Pepper** | A versatile all round flavouring (use to taste) |

## BUYING INGREDIENTS OR READY-MADE FOODS: READING THE LABELS

*Ingredients*
Labels on most packed foods must list all the ingredients. The ingredients are listed in descending order of weight at the time of their use in the preparation of the food.

*Nutritional content*
This must be given per 100 g but many labels also have information per serving. Where per serving information is given, the weight or portion size has to be stated, as in the example of a ready-made chicken curry, pictured opposite.

*Comparing meals and foods*
When comparing different meals or foods, you need to look at amount of nutrient there is per 100 g. To get an idea whether your chosen meal has a

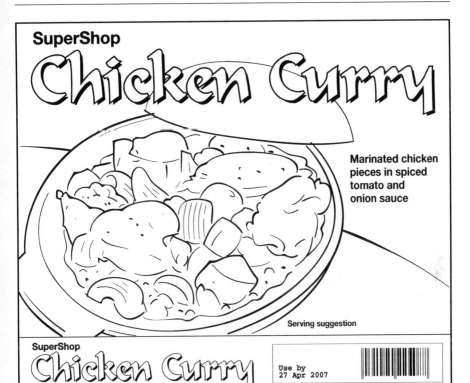

**SuperShop**

# Chicken Curry

Marinated chicken pieces in spiced tomato and onion sauce

Serving suggestion

**SuperShop**

# Chicken Curry

Use by
27 Apr 2007

## Cooking Guidelines

**Oven**
35 – 40 mins
190°C/375°F

**Microwave**
650 watt – category B 5½ mins
750 watt – category D 5 mins
850 watt – category E 4½ mins
• For best results microwave heat
• Remove outer packaging
• Pierce lid several times
• Heat on full power
• Stir well before serving

**Freezing**
• Freeze on day of purchase
• For freezing guidelines refer to manufacturer's handbook

**Oven from frozen**
45 – 50 mins
190°C/375°F
• Follow oven instructions above, adjusting heating times to 45 – 50 mins.

**Storage**
• Keep refrigerated
• Use by: see side of packet

**SuperShop**

# Chicken Curry

Marinated chicken pieces in spiced tomato and onion sauce

## Nutrition

| Typical Compos- ition | A 350g serving provides | A 100g serving provides |
|---|---|---|
| Energy | 1460kj 350kcal | 417kj 100kcal |
| Protein | 32.6g | 9.3g |
| Carbohydrate | 12.3g | 3.5g |
| of which sugars | 9.5g | 2.7g |
| Fat | 32.9g | 9.4g |
| Fibre | 5.3g | 1.5g |
| Sodium | 2.1g | 0.6g |

### 350g

Produced in the United Kingdom for
SuperShop Stores

## Ingredients

**Marinated chicken** (51%)
**Tomato** (19%)
**Onion** (7%)
**Vegetable Oil** (5.1%)
**Tomato Purée**
**Garlic Purée**
**Ginger Purée**
**Coriander**
**Chicken Stock**
**Ground Coriander**
**Onion Purée**
**Ground Cumin**
**Minced Green Chillies**
**Chicken Fat**
**Salt**

Every care has been made to remove bones, but some may still remain

lot or a little of a particular nutrient, use the 'ready reckoner' below as a guide. If you are comparing ingredients, you may also want to look at how much of that ingredient there is in the final cooked meal.

Going back to the chicken curry example, the label indicates that it contains a moderate amount of fat (9.4 g per 100 g of product) and a high level of salt (0.6 g sodium per 100 g of product).

| READY RECKONER (per 100 g of food) | |
|---|---|
| **A lot** | **A little** |
| 10.0 g sugars | 2.0 g sugars |
| 20.0 g fat | 3.0 g fat |
| 5.0 g saturates | 1.0 g saturates |
| 3.0 g fibre | 0.5 g fibre |
| 0.5 g sodium | 0.1 g sodium |

*Labelling claims*

Food labels cannot just say anything they would like to as labelling is strictly governed by law. A food cannot claim to be 'reduced calorie' unless it is much lower in calories than the usual version. Nevertheless, claims made on packaging need to be interpreted with care. This is because, with the exception of butters, margarines and other spreadable fats, the law states no legal definitions for quantities but states the claim should not be misleading and gives several recommendations.

It is useful to understand what these recommendations are to be able to compare similar foods and assess the most suitable food choice for you and your dietary goals.

- **'Reduced fat'**  When a food has a reduction claim in a nutrient (such as 'reduced fat') it is important to remember what the standard product is like to make a true assessment of the benefit of this claim. For example, we all know that pork pies are a very high-fat food. Legally, if the manufacturers reduced the fat content in the recipe by 25%, they could claim the product was 'Reduced Fat'. However, while the reduced fat option might be better than the standard product, it would still be a significant source of fat.

| Recommendations for claims on fat content | |
|---|---|
| **'Low Fat Food'** | Less than 3 g fat in 100 g of food (means the food is actually low in fat) |
| **'Reduced Fat'** | This means that the food contains three quarters (75%) of the amount of fat found in the standard equivalent |
| **'Fat free'** | Should only be used in foods that contain a tiny amount of fat (less than 0.15 g per 100 g of product) |
| **Virtually fat free** | Ambiguous: check on the nutrition panel of the label what the manufacturer actually means by this |
| **'Lite' or 'light'** | The law does not say what these terms mean, so manufacturers could convey a message about the product's texture or give the impression it has fewer calories. The label will be more informative – see what it says about nutrients per 100 g of food, as described above |

- **'Low fat'** In addition, 'low' or 'lower' in fat does not mean that the product is also low in sugar. It may even have more sugar than the original standard product. Similarly 'low in sugar' makes no claim about the fat content. There is no guarantee either that low-fat and low-sugar products are lower in calories. Often they are as high – or almost as high – in calories as the full-fat or full-sugar product.

- **'No added'** Some products carry the claim 'no added sugar (or salt)'. Again this term means that that no sugar (or salt) has been added in the manufacturing process; it does not always mean it is actually low in these nutrients. For example, we know from an average supermarket label of pure, unsweetened orange juice that a typical sugar content of 10.5 g per 100 mls means that it can still be a rich source of sugar if too much is consumed.

### Potassium and phosphate
Potassium and phosphate are rarely included in the nutritional information in the UK, so look instead at the main ingredients used. In

many cases, it is also helpful to think about how the dish or food is likely to have been cooked and prepared. You might be able to compare it with a similar dish that you make at home.

Going back to the Chicken Curry label on page 65:

- Tomatoes come second in the descending order of ingredients, which states it makes up 19 % of the weight of ingredients used. As tomatoes are relatively high in potassium, this dish is also likely to be high in potassium. If you have been asked to be careful with the amount of potassium you eat, it may not necessarily mean you can never choose this dish. But options to consider could be:
  - Choose another curry dish instead that uses less tomato
  - Choose another chicken dish such as one with a cream-based chicken sauce.

- If you do select the chicken curry as above, choose low-potassium choices to go with it (for example, plain naan bread or plain rice). Avoid dishes such as chips or Bombay potatoes where the potatoes may not have been boiled.

- If you are having the chicken curry as a treat, try reducing the amount of other foods that are high in potassium to be eaten earlier on that day, or the day after, to 'make room' for this choice.

## FOOD HYGIENE

When storing, preparing and cooking food it is always good practice to follow basic principles of food hygiene to help minimise any risk of food infection. These are some general guidelines:

- Take chilled and frozen food home quickly, then put it in your fridge or freezer promptly. Do not refreeze thawed food.

- Prepare and store raw and cooked food separately – keep raw meat and fish at the bottom of your fridge.

- Keep the coldest part of your fridge at 0–5°C. Consider buying a fridge thermometer if you don't already have one.

- Check 'use by' dates, and use food within the recommended period.

- Keep pets away from food and worktops.

- Wash your hands thoroughly before preparing food or eating.

- Wash worktops and utensils between preparing raw and cooked food.

- Do not eat foods containing uncooked eggs. Keep your eggs in the fridge.

- Cook your food well. Make sure you follow any instructions on the pack and if you reheat, ensure the food is piping hot. Do not reheat food more than once.

- Keep hot foods HOT and cold foods COLD; do not just leave them standing around.

## MEAL PLANNING

Good meal planning enables you to get the best possible balance of nutrients in the most enjoyable way, getting the taste, texture, colour and smell of the meal right as well as making sure that what you eat is good for you. We hope that reading through this book will have given you plenty of ideas about doing just this, but here are a few tips to help you make the most of the recipes. Planning meals for a restricted diet can seem a huge challenge but is really just a question of picking out the dishes that already work well for your needs, adapting others with some minor changes and perhaps introducing yourself to some new ingredients or ways of cooking.

*Classic combinations work well*
It is precisely because they work so well that they have become classics in the first place. For example:

- Bolognese sauce and pasta;
- Dahl and rice;
- Baked beans with a jacket potato.

All three provide a good balance of nutrients as well as tasting good. On the other hand, inventing new combinations can produce dishes which are just as tasty and nutritious:

- Bolognese sauce with bulgar wheat;
- Dahl with a granary roll;
- Baked beans with a chapatti or toast.

The recipes in this book have been chosen to show you how the old favourites can work well with a restricted diet and to introduce you to some new flavours, ingredients and ways of cooking. This should help to make your meals and snacks delicious, easy to prepare and fit in with any dietary changes you have been advised to make.

*Principles for a well-balanced diet*

- **Choose a starchy food for the basis of all your meals**  Potatoes and other starchy roots such as yam, plantain and sweet potato are popular choices for many of us, and a good source of energy. However, they are higher in potassium than many other starchy foods. If you need to restrict your potassium intake, boil them before eating because some of the potassium is lost into the cooking water and can then be thrown away. Use lower potassium foods – pasta, rice, bread or noodles – as alternatives.

- **Balance your nutrients**  If you are eating a food that is high in a restricted nutrient, combine it with a food that is very low in the same nutrient and you may find that the meal will fit into your diet without too great a problem. For example, if you are on a low-potassium diet, serve your lamb and okra curry with rice, bread or chapatti instead of potatoes, chips or yam. On the other hand, you may be on a low-salt diet but have a ready-made pasta sauce instead of a home-made low-salt version for convenience. In this case you could cook the pasta and any other ingredients for the meal without adding salt and salty extras such as ham or olives.

- **Be 'fluid aware'**  If you are on a fluid restriction you can also look for alternatives to gravy to moisten your food. You could try different methods of cooking meat and fish – steaming, braising, wrapping in foil – to keep in the moisture. You can gently fry the food or add some salad oil, butter, cream cheese or cream – these contain little water and are high in calories, which can also be useful if you have a small appetite and need to put on weight. For lower calorie alternatives to salty sauces try a little lemon juice, vinegar, low-fat yoghurt, cottage cheese or cream cheese. Many of the recipes in this book will give you some ideas for using these foods in your cooking.

- **Remember to eat enough fruit and vegetables**  They can be a great way to add taste, colour, texture and moisture to a meal without extra salt and fluid, as well as providing many essential vitamins, minerals and other essential nutrients. Some fruits and vegetables are high in potassium and may need to be restricted or avoided by people who have been advised to follow a low-potassium diet. They may also need to limit the total amount of fruits and vegetables eaten, but it is rare for anyone to be told to avoid them altogether. We have chosen recipes which include a variety of fruits and vegetables which are lower in potassium and which can be enjoyed by the whole family whether or not they are on a low-potassium diet.

- **Don't limit yourself** Use the information in this book and the advice from your own dietitian to adjust and adapt your favourite recipes or those in other recipe books. Many of the hints and tips in this book come from people who are following a special diet themselves and have discovered a different way to make their favourite dish taste good without adding salt or another restricted ingredient. You may not even make any of the recipes in this book but just pick up some new ideas for making your own meals and snacks taste good. We hope to make it as easy as possible for you to eat food that is both tasty and healthy. Whether reading, cooking or eating, enjoy!

# Part 2 – RECIPES

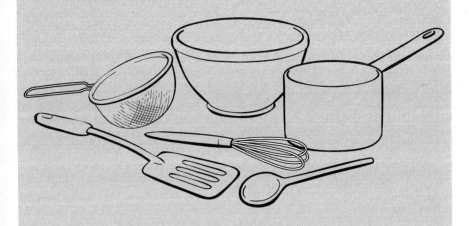

# Recipe coding

All our recipes are coded to help you choose the most suitable dishes for your dietary needs. Nutritional analysis of all recipes can be found in Appendix 2 (pages 148–9). The coding is as follows:

✳ **High energy** *Recipes with a particularly high energy content*
A complete main meal dish that provides at least 600 kcal per serving.
An incomplete main meal dish (lacking either a starch or vegetable component) or snack meal that provides at least 400 kcal per serving.
A dessert, starter or side dish providing at least 200 kcal per serving.

✳ **High protein** *Recipes with a particularly high protein content*
A main meal dish that provides at least 20 g protein per serving.
Snack meals and vegetarian dishes are coded high-protein if they provide at least 15 g per serving.
A dessert, starter or side dish that provides at least 5 g protein per serving.

✳ **Low potassium** *Suitable for inclusion in a low-potassium diet*
A complete main meal dish that provides less than 1000 mg (26 mmol) per serving.
An incomplete main dish (lacking either a starch or a vegetable component) or a snack meal that provides less than 600 mg (15 mmol) per serving.
A dessert, starter or side dish that provides less than 270 mg (7 mmol) per serving.

✳ **Low phosphate** *Suitable for inclusion in a low-phosphate diet*
A complete main meal dish that provides less than 400 mg (13 mmol) phosphorous per serving.
An incomplete main dish or snack meal that provides less than 310 mg (10 mmol) phosphorous per serving.
A dessert, starter or side dish that provides less than 150 mg (5 mmol) phosphorous per serving.

✳ **Low sodium/salt** (Not marked on individual recipes) All dishes are low in added salt and have a sodium content of below 0.5 g per 100 g.

✳ **Suitable for diabetics** *As part of a balanced, low-sugar diabetic diet*
Only desserts are coded, as it is assumed that all savoury dishes would be suitable. Dishes are not necessarily low in total fat or saturated fat. Any necessary modifications to the recipe are noted.

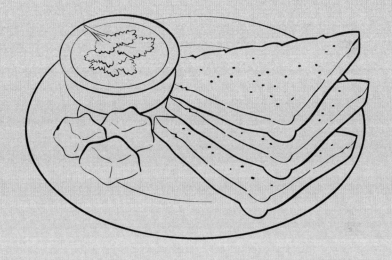

# Cheesy cheat's pizza

**Preparation time:**
10 minutes

**Cooking time:**
5–10 minutes

*A favourite midday or supper snack, this needs only a sprinkle of cheddar cheese to give you a toasted cheese flavour, which keeps the phosphate and sodium content down. If you don't think you like cottage cheese, try this dish – it may convert you.*

**Ingredients** (*serves 1*)
Wholemeal bap • 1 medium
tomato • 1 small (60 g) thinly sliced
red pepper • 2 slices (25 g)
cottage cheese • 1 generous tablespoon (50 g)
cheddar, grated • 1 tablespoon (10 g)
freshly ground black pepper • to taste
dried oregano or mixed herbs • 1 pinch (optional)

Preheat the grill to medium-high. Slice the bap in half. Lightly toast the bread on each side under a grill. Remove from the grill and top each side of the bap with slices of tomato. Sprinkle with the dried herbs if you are using them. Finely chop the red pepper and sprinkle over the tomato. Top each 'pizza' with half the cottage cheese and sprinkle evenly with the grated cheese. Return to the grill and grill until the cheddar is melted and golden brown. Serve with a little freshly ground black pepper.

### For a change
Try adding a little chopped tinned pineapple and finely chopped hot green or red chilli, or a few drops of Tabasco.

**High protein**
\*
**Low potassium**
\*
**Low phosphate**

**Cook's tip:** You could try this pizza topping on a wide range of breads including any sliced bread, rolls, pitta bread, ciabatta. Alternatively try it on homemade or bought plain pizza bases as an alternative to ready-made pizza.

# Felafel

**Preparation time:**
10 minutes

**Cooking time:**
20 minutes

*Some would call felafel the national dish of Israel and it also is popular in many other Middle Eastern countries. It is a cheap, filling and delicious vegetarian meal. This is a very easy version, made with tinned chickpeas which are good source of protein but lower in potassium and phosphate than many other beans and lentils.*

**Ingredients** *(makes 12 felafel balls or 4 servings)*
tinned chickpeas • 1 can (approx 450 g), drained
onion • 1 small, chopped
fresh parsley leaves • 2 tablespoons
garlic • 1 clove, crushed
egg • 1
dried coriander • 1 teaspoon
dried cumin • 1 teaspoon
black pepper • freshly ground
dried breadcrumbs or matzo meal • 45 g
vegetable oil • for frying

*To serve*
pitta breads • 2
crème fraîche or natural yoghurt • 150 g
carrot • 1 small, grated
cucumber • 10 cm chunk, grated

Place the chickpeas, onion, parsley, garlic, egg and spices in a large bowl. Use a hand blender to mix and process the mixture until the chickpeas are blended but not puréed. This can also be done in a food processor.

Add enough of the breadcrumbs until the mixture forms a small ball without sticking to your hands. Form the chickpea mixture into 12 balls and flatten slightly. Heat the oil in a frying pan and cook the felafels over a medium heat, turning over once during cooking, until golden brown on both sides. Drain on a paper towel. Lightly toast pitta breads, split and fill each half with three felafels. Mix the grated carrot and cucumber together and divide between the pitta breads. Drizzle with the crème fraîche or yoghurt.

**High protein**
✳
**Low potassium**
✳
**Low phosphate**

**SNACKS AND STARTERS**

# Flavoured 'butters'

**Preparation time:**
10 minutes

**Cooking time:**
none

**Chilling time:**
30 minutes minimum

*This is a version of a catering classic, ideal for adding difference to a meal. Try spreading the 'butters' on bread, crackers or even use them as a topping for boiled potatoes, vegetables, grilled meat or fish. It can be a great way to liven up a simple dish.*

*We have substituted a healthier, salt-free margarine for the traditional butter, which also reduces the sodium content. You could also choose a reduced-fat margarine if you prefer a lower-fat option.*

**Ingredients** *(makes 6 small portions)*
unsalted olive oil-/sunflower-based margarine • 50 g

### IDEAS FOR ADDITIONS:

**Lemon and parsley margarine**
fresh parsley • 2 tablespoons chopped
lemon • grated zest and juice of half

**Chilli and lime margarine**
fresh red chilli • half, de-seeded and finely diced
lime • grated zest and juice of half

Leave the margarine out of the fridge for 15 minutes, as this will make the mixing easier. Place in a small mixing bowl, add in your choice of flavours and blend well together. Return to the fridge for at least 30 minutes to harden. When needed, place in a small dish for serving or use as suggested above. Alternatively, you could slice the 'butter' into portions or use a melon baller to form a ball shape for an attractive accompaniment to warm fresh bread.

**Low potassium**
✳
**Low phosphate**

# Pitta crisps with tzatziki dip

Preparation time:
5 minutes

Cooking time:
20 minutes

*It can be hard to find savoury biscuits, crackers or crisps that you can eat on a low-potassium or low-salt diet. These crisps are easy to make, are surprisingly moreish and will keep for a few days in an airtight container.*

## Ingredients
*(makes about 24 crisps or about 8 servings)*

### For the crisps
pitta breads • 4
olive oil • 2 tablespoons
black pepper, freshly ground

### For the tzatziki dip
low-fat plain yoghurt • 1 small pot (150 g)
mint sauce • 1 teaspoon
cucumber • 5 cm slice (approx 70 g), finely diced

Preheat the oven to 170°C (Gas Mark 3). Brush each pitta bread on both sides with olive oil. Tear or cut each pitta breads into about 6 pieces and spread out on a baking tray. Sprinkle black pepper over the pitta bread pieces. Bake for about 20 minutes or until crisp and lightly browned. Leave to cool on a wire rack.

High protein
＊
Low potassium
＊
Low phosphate

### For a change
You can experiment with some different flavoured pitta crisps by using your favourite dried herbs or spices. We like a sprinkle of garam masala, or dried oregano.

**SNACKS AND STARTERS**

# Stilton spread with Melba toast

**Preparation time:**
10 minutes

**Cooking time:**
5–10 minutes

*Stilton is high in sodium and phosphate, so you may be missing it if you are on a restricted diet. This recipe uses cream cheese flavoured with Stilton for an easy starter idea. It will give you a taste of Stilton but less of the phosphate and sodium. You could also use the mixture as a sandwich filling. Melba toast is an easy, low-potassium, low-phosphate snack; a 1970s classic that deserves a comeback.*

**Ingredients** *(serves 4)*
cream cheese • 150 g
Stilton • 20 g
black pepper • to taste
bread • 2 thin slices from a ready-cut,
      brown or white loaf

In a mixing bowl beat the two cheeses together until well blended. Add 1–2 teaspoons of milk if you prefer a thinner consistency. Remove crusts from bread and toast lightly.

Using a bread knife, carefully split the slices through the middle and toast the uncooked surfaces under a hot grill until crisp and brown. Serve a scoop of Stilton spread with a slice of Melba toast.

**Cook's tip:** This goes well with a few leaves of watercress or rocket salad or a couple of slices of fresh or tinned pear, depending on your dietary restrictions and preferences

High energy
✳
Low potassium
✳
Low phosphate

**Hint:** Use low-fat cream cheese to decrease the fat and calorie content of this dish.

# Tuna pâté

**Preparation time:**
10 minutes

**Cooking time:**
None

*Pâté made in the traditional way, with liver, is high in phosphate. This recipe is lower in phosphate and also works well as a option for non-meat eaters. You can use this pâté as a dip with toast, or as a regular sandwich filling.*

**Ingredients** *(topping for 4 toasts)*
tuna • 200 g tin in springwater, drained
lemon • half, squeezed
fresh parsley • 1 tablespoon, chopped
fresh dill • 1 tablespoon, chopped
       (or 1 teaspoon dried dill)
dill pickle • 1 medium, diced
olive oil • 1 teaspoon
mayonnaise • 1 teaspoon
wholemeal toast • 4 slices

**High protein**
✳
**Low potassium**
✳
**Low phosphate**

Mix the tuna, lemon juice, parsley, dill, olive oil and mayonnaise and then add to a food processor. Whizz together for a minute until texture is smooth – this can be reduced or increased to taste. Remove the mixture from the food processor and stir in the diced pickle. Serve with the toast.

    This recipe can also be made in a bowl and blended using a hand blender.

# SANDWICH IDEAS

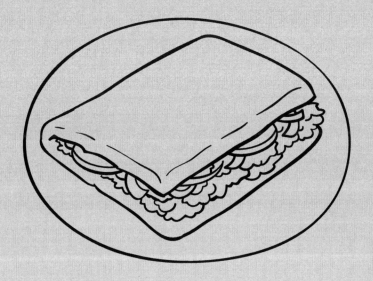

# A fresh look at bread and sandwiches

A sandwich makes a quick and easy meal and can be just as nutritious as a cooked meal. Eating more sandwiches can be a good way to overcome a poor appetite. By adding extra butter, margarine or mayonnaise to your sandwich you can give yourself a high-calorie boost to put on weight. On the other hand, you can make your sandwich high in fibre and low in fat to help you lose some weight or just to help you eat more healthily.

## Some of the wide variety of breads available

| | |
|---|---|
| Brown | White sliced |
| Granary | Wholemeal |
| Chapatti | Rye |
| French bread | English muffin |
| Soft granary bap | Crusty white roll |
| Tortilla wrap | Pitta bread |
| Bagel | Croissant |
| Naan | Ciabatta |

## HOME BREADMAKING

If you make your own bread, try reducing the amount of salt you add. You will probably find that you can cut the salt added in a standard recipe by as much as half to make a loaf that tastes just as good. Adding flavourings such as cinnamon, dried or fresh herbs, garlic and onion are a good way to add taste and variety to your homemade bread.

# Tasty sandwich fillings

For variety, try some of these ideas and combinations.

**Beef and mustard**
Thick slices of bread from a crusty white loaf, spread with English mustard and filled with cold roast beef.

**Chicken and mango**
Cold, shredded roast chicken with 1 teaspoon mango chutney in wholemeal pitta.

**Cottage cheese and peach on an English muffin**
Toast and split an English muffin. Spread each side with a tablespoon of cottage cheese and top with slices of tinned peach. Sprinkle with a pinch of cinnamon and a teaspoon of brown sugar and place under a hot grill until the sugar bubbles.

**Houmous bagel**
Houmous and a little grated carrot in a toasted bagel.

**Lamb and mint**
Spread the roll or bread with mint sauce and fill with cold roast lamb.

**Mexican chicken mix**
Cold diced roast chicken, mixed with sour cream or mayonnaise, a little diced red pepper and a few drops of Tabasco sauce.

**Tuna mix**
Tinned tuna (tinned in spring water if possible), mixed with mayonnaise and a small pickled cucumber, finely chopped – good in a granary roll.

**Tuna and mustard**
Tinned tuna (in spring water if possible) mixed with a little olive oil and wholegrain mustard to taste.

**Turkey and cranberry sauce (Thanksgiving tortilla)**
Cranberry sauce is low in potassium and is a traditional accompaniment to turkey for Thanksgiving in the USA. Try in thickly sliced wholemeal bread or spread the cranberry sauce on a warmed tortilla wrap, add some shredded cold roast turkey and some crispy lettuce, and roll up.

SANDWICH IDEAS

## Cottage and cream cheese cheaters

We often recommend using cream cheese and cottage cheese, as they are low in phosphate and sodium. Standard cream cheese is high in fat and is ideal if you are trying to eat a high-energy diet. If you want to limit the amount of fat you eat, or are trying to lose weight, you can use low-fat cream cheese or cottage cheese. Unfortunately many people tell us that they find cottage and cream cheese boring or tasteless. Luckily there are many flavoured varieties of these cheeses – you can buy them mixed with herbs, garlic, pineapple and lots more. Another approach is to use cottage and cream cheese to 'stretch' a small amount of foods which are higher in phosphate or sodium such as hard cheeses or bacon. This gives you more flavour than plain cream or cottage cheese and allows you to enjoy a taste of the restricted food.

Try adding any of the following to plain cream cheese or cottage cheese:

Tinned pineapple or peaches, chopped or sliced
Finely diced red pepper, grated carrot or cooked frozen peas
A small slice of crispy bacon, crumbled
A small slice of smoked salmon, finely chopped
Tinned tuna, flaked
Pickled cucumber, finely chopped
Fresh herbs, finely chopped – e.g. parsley, thyme, dill, coriander
Mango chutney
Cinnamon powder
Fresh or pickled chillis, finely sliced

## To add salad – or not?

If you are on a low-potassium diet and restrict the amount of vegetables you eat, you will have to include any salad in this restriction. In most cases a small amount of salad in a sandwich can be taken in addition or instead of your normal vegetable or fruit allowance. Ask your dietitian for advice if you are unsure about including salad in your sandwich.

# A trio of toasts

### Cinnamon toast
Preheat the grill to medium. Toast a slice of bread on one side only. Spread the untoasted side with butter or margarine. Sprinkle with a mixture of 1 teaspoon of caster sugar and 1–2 generous pinches of ground cinnamon (or mixed spice). Grill until the toast is browned at the edges. Allow to cool slightly before eating as the sugar can get very hot. Eat alone as an afternoon snack or for breakfast. Also try with fresh or tinned fruit or plain cottage cheese. The sugar-spice mixture can be made in larger quantities and kept in an airtight container.

### Garlic toast
Preheat the grill to medium. Toast a slice of bread on one side only. Peel and crush a small garlic clove and mix with 3 tsp (or more) olive oil. Spread the untoasted side with the garlic oil . Grill until lightly browned. Sprinkle with finely chopped fresh herbs if liked. Good with meat stews as a low-potassium alternative to potatoes. Also goes well with omelettes, scrambled egg and many other savoury dishes.

### French toast ('eggy bread')
Beat one egg with a tablespoon of milk in a shallow dish. Place a slice of bread in the egg mixture, making sure that the side in the egg is completely coated. Turn the bread over and leave for at least 5 minutes or until most or all the egg had soaked into the bread. Prick the bread with a fork several times to allow more egg to be soaked up. Heat a little fat or oil in a frying pan and over a medium heat cook the bread slice on both sides until browned. Serve immediately alone or with a sprinkle of cheese or cinnamon or cinnamon sugar (see above). This makes a tasty and nutritious breakfast or light lunch or supper, particularly for someone with a small appetite.

SANDWICH IDEAS

# FISH DISHES

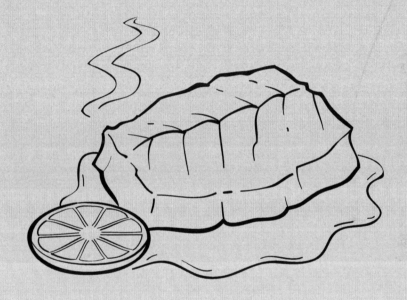

# Crispy tangy fish

Preparation time:
25 minutes

Cooking time:
30 minutes

*White fish such as cod, haddock and plaice are high in protein, and this is a way to give these good old favourites a different taste. The recipe includes some salty ingredients but the amounts used are small and no further salt needs to be added.*

**Ingredients** *(serves 2)*
cod fillets • 2 medium
unsalted margarine or butter • 15 g
plain flour • 2 rounded tablespoons
lemon juice • 1 tablespoon
semi-skimmed milk • 150 mls
fresh breadcrumbs • 25 g
mature cheddar cheese • 25 g, grated
bacon • 25 g, chopped and rind removed
chopped parsley • to garnish
pepper • to taste

Preheat the oven to 190°C/Gas Mark 5. Place the fish fillets in a shallow ovenproof dish. Combine the breadcrumbs, bacon and cheese in a bowl.

Next, make the white sauce. Melt the margarine in a saucepan and stir in the flour. Gradually blend in the milk, stirring all the time. As the sauce thickens add in the lemon juice and pepper and remove from the heat.

Pour the sauce over the fish fillets and sprinkle the breadcrumb mixture over the sauce. Bake in the preheated oven for 30 minutes. If you like, you can garnish with the chopped parsley just before serving.

**High protein**

# Crunchy olive and lime plaice

**Preparation time:**
25 minutes

**Cooking time:**
30 minutes

*This also works well with any other white fish such as cod or haddock, These are all good sources of protein and low in fat and phosphate. A handy way to make the breadcrumbs is to toast a slice of wholemeal bread well, and leave to stand for a few minutes, after which it can be crumbled into small pieces.*

**Ingredients** *(serves 2)*
plaice fillets • 2
garlic • 2 cloves, crushed
green olives • 6–7, stoned and finely chopped
fresh wholemeal breadcrumbs • 30 g (see above)
lime • zest of half, and juice of one
olive oil • 2 tablespoons
fresh parsley • 1 tablespoon, chopped
pepper • to taste

Preheat the oven to 200°C (Gas Mark 6). Place the fish in a lightly greased shallow ovenproof dish and evenly spread the oil and about three quarters of the lime juice on top of it. Place in the oven and cook for 25 minutes, occasionally basting the fish by spooning over any of the juices in the dish.

**High protein**

✳

**Low potassium**

✳

**Low phosphate**

While the fish is cooking, mix together all the other remaining ingredients. Once cooking has finished, remove from the fish from the oven and spread the crunchy olive mixture evenly on top of each plaice fillet. Return to the oven for a further 5 minutes and serve once the crumb topping is golden.

# Fish steaks with orange, lemon and mustard

**Preparation time:**
15 minutes
plus marinating time

**Cooking time:**
6 minutes, microwave;
16–20 minutes, grill

*This dish works well with salmon or any of the white fish which are lower in phosphate. The citrus fruits and mustard add plenty of flavour so no extra salt is needed. It is a great dish for entertaining or as after-work supper as it is best prepared the day before and left to marinate overnight to help develop the flavours. If prepared on the same day, try to allow at least two hours for marinating.*

**Ingredients** *(serves 2)*
salmon or white fish • 2 medium steaks or fillets
lemon • zest of half and juice of one
orange • zest of half and juice of one
olive oil • 1 tablespoon
wholegrain mustard • 1 tablespoon
chopped dill • 1 tablespoon (fresh if possible)
pepper • to taste

Score across each salmon steak 2–3 times to allow greater penetration of the marinade. Mix together the citrus zest, juice, olive oil, mustard and dill. Place the fish in a microwaveable dish with the flesh part facing downwards. Add the citrus mixture, ensuring the fish is well covered. Leave to marinate overnight.

When you are ready to cook, microwave the fish in the marinade on high for 6 minutes. Serve with a little of the marinade. If you don't have a microwave, place the fish under a medium grill for 8–10 minutes on each side, or until it is cooked through.

**High protein**
❊
**Low potassium**
❊
**Low phosphate**

### Serving suggestion
This dish goes well with the garlic and herb mashed potatoes, on page 127.

# Plaice with a creamy coriander topping

**Preparation time:**
10 minutes

**Cooking time:**
5–10 minutes

*A great way to cook any fairly thin piece of fish, especially for anyone on a fluid restriction as it makes the fish moist without adding any extra sauce.*

**Ingredients** *(serves 2)*
plaice fillets • 2 (approx 250 g in total)
cream cheese • 70 g
lemon juice • 1 teaspoon
coriander leaves • 2 tablespoons, finely chopped, fresh
black pepper • to taste

Lay the place fillets on a lightly oiled baking tray. Mix the remaining ingredients together. Dividing the cheese mixture into two portions, spread each portion over the top of the plaice. Chill in the fridge for about 10 minutes to firm the mixture.

Preheat the grill to high. Grill the plaice without turning for approximately 5 minutes or until cooked through.

Try serving with some boiled new potatoes and boiled broccoli.

**High protein**
✳
**Low potassium**
✳
**Low phosphate**

**Cook's tip:** A delicious variation of this recipe can be made by using 2 teaspoons of wholegrain mustard instead of the herbs.

**Hint:** Use low-fat cream cheese to reduce the calorie and fat content of this dish.

# Thai tuna fishcakes

Preparation time:
20 minutes
and 15 minutes
chilling time

Cooking time:
10–20 minutes
(depending on
the size of your pan)

*You can try this recipe with any tinned or cooked fish such as salmon, cod, whiting or mackerel. Cook the potatoes by boiling in plenty of water to remove some potassium if you are on a low-potassium diet.*

**Ingredients** *(serves 2 as a main course)*
cooked, mashed potatoes • 250 g
unsalted margarine or butter • 15 g
tinned tuna • 250 g drained weight
green chilli • 1 small, finely chopped
fresh coriander • 1 tablespoon (15 g)
small lime • juice and grated zest
plain flour • approx 1 tablespoon
vegetable oil • for frying
mangetout peas • 150 g

Place the potatoes in a bowl and beat in the tuna, chilli, coriander and lime zest. Add the lime juice and zest to make a soft but firm mixture. Divide the mixture into six equal portions and, with floured hands, form each into a flat cake. Lightly coat each fishcake in flour and chill in the fridge for at least 15 minutes (or overnight) to firm up.

Heat the oil in a frying pan over a medium heat. Then fry the fishcakes for about 5 minutes on each side or until nicely browned. Drain on kitchen paper and serve while still hot with the freshly drained mangetout peas.

### Serving suggestion
Instead of the mangetout, you could serve with boiled peas or another boiled vegetable of your choice. If you are on a potassium restriction, avoid serving with extra potatoes but plain or flavoured rice would be a good alternative (see page 128). The Thai fishcakes are also good served with a crispy salad and some pitta bread.

High protein
❋
Low potassium
❋
Low phosphate

**Cook's tip:** If you prefer a less exotic taste to your fishcakes, leave out the coriander, lime and chilli and instead use 1 tablespoon of fresh parsley, zest and juice of half a lemon and ground pepper to taste.

# Tuna pasta Niçoise

**Preparation time:**
20 minutes

**Cooking time:**
20 minutes

*This versatile dish can be served as a main meal or as a snack or starter. Pasta is a good source of energy and the tuna provides high-quality protein. The vegetables should be included within your potassium allowance if you are on a low-potassium diet.*

**Ingredients** *(serves 2 as a meal or 4 as a starter)*
dried pasta shapes (e.g. bows/farfalle) • 130 g
French beans • 100 g
Dijon mustard • 1 teaspoon
vinegar • 2 tablespoons
olive oil • 4 tablespoons
tuna steak, canned in oil • 200 g tin, drained
fresh basil • 1 heaped tablespoons, chopped
black olives • 10, chopped in half lengthways
egg • 1 boiled, sliced into quarters

Boil the pasta, drain and allow to cool to room temperature. Top and tail the French beans; cut in half and boil until tender. Drain and allow to cool.

To make the French dressing, mix together the olive oil, mustard, basil and vinegar, adding pepper to taste.

In a serving dish combine the pasta, beans, tuna in bite size chunks and the olives. Mix in the French dressing and serve with the quartered egg on top.

**High energy**
*
**High protein**
*
**Low potassium**
*
**Low phosphate**

**Hint:** Add more or less oil to increase or decrease the energy (calorie) content of a dish.

**FISH DISHES**

# Tuna steaks with caramelised balsamic shallots

**Preparation time:**
15 minutes

*Fresh tuna is a low-fat fish which is low in phosphate. It is also a source of omega-3 fish oils, which are good for the heart.*

**Cooking time:**
10–15 minutes

**Ingredients** *(serves 4)*
fresh tuna steaks • 4 (approximately 500 g total)
rapeseed or sunflower oil • 1 tablespoon
shallots • 4, peeled and sliced
balsamic vinegar • 100 mls
lemon • grated zest and juice of half
pepper • to taste

Grill the tuna steak under a moderate heat for 10–15 minutes, turning occasionally.

**High protein**
✳
**Low potassium**
✳
**Low phosphate**

While the tuna is cooking, heat the oil in a frying pan and cook the shallots. Once they are golden brown, add the balsamic vinegar, lemon juice and zest. Bring to the boil to thicken slightly.

When the fish is cooked thoroughly, remove from the grill, top with the caramelised onions and serve immediately.

# MEAT AND POULTRY

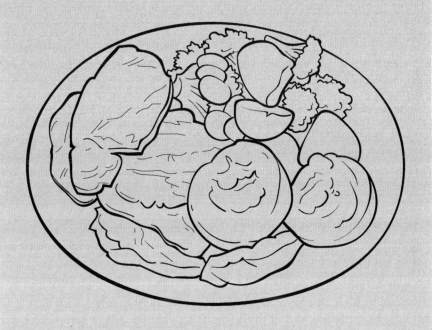

# Beef and mushroom stroganoff

**Preparation time:**
30 minutes
(including cooking
time)

*Traditional stroganoff usually contains tomatoes, but this version uses mustard instead to reduce the potassium content while still providing plenty of flavour. We have also used tinned mushrooms instead of fresh ones as they are much lower in potassium.*

**Ingredients** *(serves 4)*
stewing beef • 500 g, cut into small strips
sliced mushrooms • 1 small tin, drained
wholegrain mustard • 4 heaped teaspoons
crème fraîche • 1 (200 ml) tub
onion • 1 small, thinly sliced
rapeseed or sunflower oil • 10 ml
white wine • 150 ml
white rice • 220 g

**High energy**
✻
**High protein**
✻
**Low potassium**
✻
**Low phosphate**

Heat the oil in a pan and fry the onions until they are clear and softened. Add in the beef strips and fry for a further 5 minutes. Next add the wine and the mushrooms, cover the pan and let the mixture simmer for about 15 minutes. Meanwhile, boil the rice in unsalted water.

When the beef is evenly cooked, add the mustard and crème fraîche, and warm through before serving with the boiled rice.

# Carnival chicken with peppers and rice

**Preparation time:**
15 minutes

**Cooking time:**
1 hour

*A very flavoursome and colourful dish, which is easy to cook too. Using chopped tomatoes drained of their juice keeps the potassium content down. Rice is the perfect low-potassium accompaniment to this recipe.*

**Ingredients** *(serves 4)*
chicken portions on the bone
   (e.g. thighs) • 4–8 (about 650 g in total)
olive oil • 1 tablespoon
dry white wine • 150 ml
lemon • juice of half
boiling water • 250 ml
hot pepper sauce • 1 teaspoon
basmati rice • 250 g
onion • 1 medium, chopped
yellow pepper • 1 medium, chopped
red pepper • 1 medium, chopped
chopped tomatoes • 400 g tin, drained

Preheat the oven to 200°C (Gas Mark 6).
   Place the chicken in an ovenproof dish and coat with the olive oil and ground black pepper. Cover and cook in the oven for 20 minutes.
   Remove the chicken from the dish and add the chopped onion and peppers. Mix the wine, water, hot pepper sauce and lemon juice and add to the dish. Stir in the chopped tomatoes and rice.
   Place the chicken on top of the mixture, cover and return to the oven for a further 40 minutes or until all of the liquid has been taken up by rice.

**Cook's tip 1:** Vary the amount of hot pepper sauce to suit your taste preferences.

High protein
✳
Low potassium
✳
Low phosphate

**Cook's tip 2:** If you don't like your chicken on the bone, this dish could also be made with chicken breast portions.

# Chicken and mushroom pastry parcels

**Preparation time:**
20 minutes

**Cooking time:**
30–45 minutes

*This is a quick main course dish using pastry, a high-calorie food that is low in potassium and phosphate. The parcels could also be eaten cold for a picnic or packed lunch, making a change from sandwiches. Although fresh mushrooms are high in potassium, canned mushrooms are not, and are delicious in combination with the chicken.*

**Ingredients** *(serves 4)*
sunflower oil • 2 tablespoons
small onion • 1 finely chopped
garlic • 1 clove, crushed
dried mixed herbs • 1 teaspoon
sliced mushrooms • 1 small tin, drained
cooked chicken • 225 g (white or dark meat)
cream cheese • 100 g
ready-made shortcrust pastry • 500 g pack

Preheat the oven to 200° C / Gas Mark 6.

In a large frying pan, gently fry the onion in the oil until softened. Stir in the crushed garlic. Drain the mushrooms and stir into the onion mixture with the diced chicken meat and the herbs.

Remove from the heat, stir in the cream cheese and leave to cool.

On a floured surface, roll the pastry into a rectangle approximately 30 cm x 40 cm and cut into four rectangles. Divide the chicken mixture into four and spread over the pastry, leaving a 1 cm border. Brush the edges of the pastry squares with water and fold over to make a parcel. Pinch edges together firmly to seal in the filling. Transfer to a lightly greased baking sheet and brush with beaten egg or milk.

Bake for 30–40 minutes until golden. Serve with freshly boiled mixed vegetables such as cauliflower, peas, carrots or a mixed green salad.

**High energy**
✳
**High protein**
✳
**Low potassium**
✳
**Low phosphate**

**Cook's tip:** Instead of the dried mixed herbs, you can use your favourite herbs such as fresh or dried parsley, oregano, tarragon etc.

# Chicken with capers

Preparation time:
30 minutes

Cooking time:
1 hour

*This is chicken Italian-style but without the usual large amount of tomatoes that the Italians often love. It is low in fat but full of flavour and is delicious served with pasta, a low-potassium alternative to potato.*

## Ingredients *(serves 4)*
chicken breasts • 4 small, skinnned
olive oil • 4 tablespoons
onion • ½ medium, finely chopped
garlic cloves • 2, crushed
green pepper • 1, seeded and cut into large chunks
sliced mushrooms • 1 small tin (160 g drained weight)
chopped tomatoes • 1 large tin (400 g approx)
dry white wine • 150 ml
black pepper • to taste
capers • 2 tablespoons
tagliatelli or other dried pasta • 240 g

Preheat the oven to 180°C (Gas Mark 4). Heat the oil in a frying pan and fry the chicken breasts until browned all over. Remove from the pan and place in an ovenproof casserole dish. Add the onion to the pan and soften over a gentle heat. Add the garlic and the peppers and cook for a further 2 minutes. Drain the tomatoes, discarding the juice, and add to the pan with the mushrooms. Spread the vegetable mixture over the chicken. Pour over the wine, season with black pepper and cover the casserole tightly.

Cook in the oven for 1 hour or until the chicken is very tender. Add the capers to the dish and stir briefly.

Serve with the tagliatelli, boiled in unsalted water.

**Cook's tip 1:** If you are cooking for fewer than four people, this dish keeps well overnight in the fridge. If you reheat food, make sure that it is piping hot all the way through and do not reheat more than once.

High protein
✳

Low potassium
✳

Low phosphate

**Cook's tip 2:** Draining the tinned tomatoes and using tinned instead of fresh mushrooms reduces the potassium content of the dish.

MEAT AND POULTRY

# Chilli burgers with two relishes

Preparation time:
10 minutes

Cooking time:
15 minutes

*Shop-bought burgers are usually very high in salt. So it is handy to have a quick and easy recipe to make yourself. For alternatives to the burger bun, try pitta bread, ciabatta, granary bap, rice or couscous.*

**Ingredients** *(makes 4 burgers)*
lean minced beef • 250 g
wholemeal bread • 1 slice
semi-skimmed milk • 50 mls
chilli powder • 1 ½ teaspoons
garlic • 1 clove, crushed
hamburger buns • 4, lightly toasted or warmed

Add the milk to the bread and let it soak for a couple of minutes. Break up the moistened bread in to small pieces and add the minced beef, chilli powder, garlic and mix well. Form into four burgers and place these under the grill for about 15 minutes until they are well cooked. Serve in hamburger buns with the two relishes below.

**For Sour Cream Relish mix together:**
soured cream • 75 mls
pickled cucumber • 1 medium, finely diced
small chilli pepper • 1 fresh, seeds removed, finely diced
(*or* 1 teaspoon finely diced Jalapeno pepper)

**For Red Pepper Relish mix together:**
red pepper • quarter, diced
spring onion • 1, finely sliced
fresh coriander • 1 tablespoon, chopped
olive oil • 1 tablespoon
vinegar • 1 tablespoon

High protein
✳
Low potassium
✳
Low phosphate

*Cook's tip*
For a herby variation, instead of the chilli powder try altering the burger seasoning to 2 tablespoons basil and 2 tablespoons oregano.

# Garlic chicken

**Preparation time:**
10 minutes

**Cooking time:**
1 hour

*This is a one-pot recipe, which requires little culinary skill and is a very aromatic dish. The garlic gives plenty of taste without the need for any salt or other sauce. Ideal when served with rice, pasta or potatoes. However, not recommended for romantic evenings!*

**Ingredients** *(serves 4)*
chicken portions on the bone
   (e.g. thighs) • 4–8 (about 650 g in total)
garlic • 1 bulb (6 cloves)
olive oil • 2 tablespoons
courgette • 1 medium (approx 80 g), cubed
red pepper • ½ medium (approx 80 g)
green pepper • ½ medium (approx 80 g)

Pre-heat the oven to 220°C (Gas Mark 7).

On the hob, heat the oil in an ovenproof dish and add the finely chopped garlic. Cook over a low heat for 2–3 minutes but do not allow to burn. As the garlic begins to brown, add the courgette, the peppers and the chicken quarters. Toss in the garlicky oil ensuring that all the ingredients are well coated and the chicken is sealed.

Move the dish to the oven and cook for approximately 1 hour. Check that the chicken is cooked by pricking with a fork to see if the juices run clear.

**High protein**
✳
**Low potassium**
✳
**Low phosphate**

### Cook's tip
Use less garlic for a more subtle flavour.

# Grilled marinated chicken

**Preparation time:**
15 minutes
plus marinating time

**Cooking time:**
15 minutes

*This is a way to flavour your chicken and keep it moist without needing gravy. Soya sauce is very high in salt but you should be able to find low-sodium soya sauce in most supermarkets. To get the best flavours from this dish, marinate the chicken overnight, or at least for a few hours. The chicken can be grilled as below or cubed and served as a kebab option on a barbecue.*

**Ingredients** *(serves 2)*
chicken breast fillets • 2 (approx 260 g total)
low-sodium (salt) soy sauce • 2 tablespoons
sherry • 4 tablespoons
honey • 1 tablespoon
sesame oil • 1 tablespoon

Slice the chicken breasts in half horizontally so that the two halves open to make a heart shape. This will make grilling easier.

Mix together the soy sauce, honey, sherry and sesame oil and spoon over the chicken. Leave to marinate for at least 30 minutes or overnight.

When you want to start cooking, remove the chicken from the marinade, discard remaining marinade and grill the chicken for about 15 minutes.

**High protein**

✳

**Low potassium**

✳

**Low phosphate**

Serve when it is thoroughly cooked.

### Serving suggestion
This dish goes well with rice, noodles or boiled potatoes.

# Lamb boulangère

**Preparation time:**
20 minutes

**Cooking time:**
90 minutes approx

*This classic dish originated with the Greeks, who used to prepare the dish at home but get the village bakers to cook it in their bread ovens.*

*Pre-boiling the potatoes helps to keep the potassium content of this dish low. Equally, using water with bay leaves, garlic and thyme rather than the traditional stock, keeps the salt content low without reducing flavour.*

**Ingredients** *(serves 4)*
leg or boned shoulder of lamb • 500 g
garlic • 2 cloves, finely chopped
onion • 1 medium, peeled and quartered
potatoes • 500 g, peeled and cut into small chunks
thyme • 1 tablespoon
bay leaves • 2
olive oil • 2 tablespoons
pepper • to season
water • 150 ml
carrots • 150 g, peeled and finely sliced
frozen green peas • 150 g

Pre-heat the oven to 200° C (Gas Mark 6). Rub the garlic into the lamb. Boil the potato for 10 minutes, then drain.

Meanwhile, use a little of the oil to oil the ovenproof dish. Finely chop the onion, thyme and bay leaves, and mix with the potato pieces and remaining oil. Place the potato mixture in the dish. Season with a little freshly ground pepper, cover the potatoes with the boiling water and bake for 30 minutes.

Check regularly to prevent the potatoes drying out and add a little more water if necessary. Place the lamb on the mixture and return to the oven for an hour, a little longer if you like your meat well done. Allow the meat to stand for 15 minutes before carving. Boil the carrots and peas in unsalted water and serve with the meat.

You can adapt this recipe for cooking pork or chicken.

**High protein**
*
**Low potassium**
*
**Low phosphate**

# Pork with a honey and mustard glaze

**Preparation time:**
5 minutes

**Cooking time:**
20 minutes

*This is an easy and quick dinner suggestion which requires a minimum of preparation time. The glaze adds flavour and keeps the meat moist, so there is no need for salty gravy. This is handy if the amount of salt and/or fluid you can take is limited. If you have diabetes, you may wish to reduce the quantity of honey in the recipe by half. If you prefer a stronger mustard flavour, substitute the wholegrain with English mustard.*

**Ingredients** *(serves 2)*
pork chops • 2 medium
honey • 4 teaspoons
wholegrain mustard • 1 teaspoon
chopped parsley • for decoration

Place the pork chops under the grill and turn them intermittently for about 20 minutes or until they are thoroughly cooked. If your chops are thick, you may want to score them 2–3 times to help cooking.

While the chops are grilling, mix together the honey and mustard. When the chops are ready, serve on a plate and put 2 teaspoons of the honey and mustard mix on each. Garnish with the parsley.

**High energy**
✳
**High protein**
✳
**Low potassium**
✳
**Low phosphate**

### Serving suggestion
This dish goes well with plain boiled or mashed potatoes or rice. Alternatively, try the cheesy mash recipe on page 127.

# Pork with basil and egg noodles

**Preparation time:**
15 minutes

**Cooking time:**
10 minutes

*A quick and tasty stir-fry in true 'fusion cuisine' style. The olive oil, pine nuts and basil give this Chinese-style stir-fry an almost Italian flavour. Normally, nuts would be avoided if you were following a low-potassium diet. However, using them in small amounts and in combination with the egg noodles keeps the potassium and phosphate levels down.*

**Ingredients** *(serves 4)*
pork tenderloin • 400 g, cut in to thin strips
olive oil • 2 tablespoons
dried egg noodles • 250 g
onion • 1 medium (approx 150 g) finely sliced
balsamic vinegar • 2 tablespoons
fresh basil • 40 g, chopped coarsely
pine nuts • 1 tablespoon

Cook the noodles in accordance with the instructions on the packet. Drain off any excess water and toss the noodles with a little olive oil.

Heat a wok until very hot; add the olive oil and swirl it around and allow it the coat the wok. Add the strips of pork and fry for 2 or 3 minutes. Add in the onion and fry for a further 1 or 2 minutes. Add in the chopped basil, the balsamic vinegar and pine nuts. Mix well, ensuring that the basil and pine nuts are well coated with oil before mixing in the noodles. Mix well once more, drizzle with a little more of the olive oil if you like, and then serve.

**High protein**
٭
**Low potassium**
٭
**Low phosphate**

### Cook's tip
This dish also works well with chicken.

# Pork with caramelised apple and crème fraîche

**Preparation time:**
15 minutes

**Cooking time:**
20 minutes

*Pork and apple is a classic combination. In this version the crème fraîche makes a creamy, delicious sauce. You may find crème fraîche is a useful addition to other similar dishes as it is low in phosphate and salt, especially if you need extra calories to boost your energy intake. If not, low-fat versions are available.*

**Ingredients** *(serves 2)*
pork chops • 2 medium
granny smith apple • 1 medium, cored and sliced
crème fraîche • 100 ml
onion • 1 small, sliced
rapeseed or sunflower oil • 1 teaspoon

Place the pork chops under a preheated grill (200° C) turning them intermittently for about 20 minutes until they are thoroughly cooked.

While the chops are cooking, brown the onions with the oil in a frying pan for 5 minutes. When these are golden, add the sliced apple and cook for another 5 minutes until tender. Add the crème fraîche and keep on a low heat until the mixture has warmed up.

Serve the cooked pork on a plate and spoon over the apple and crème fraîche sauce.

**High energy**
✳

**High protein**
✳

**Low potassium**
✳

**Low phosphate**

### Serving suggestion
Try boiled rice or rosemary-flavoured potatoes with this dish.

### Cook's tip
The fat content of this dish can be reduced by trimming all the fat and rind off the pork chop, and choosing reduced-fat crème fraîche.

# Tandoori-style kebabs

Preparation time:
20 minutes, plus
1 hour minimum
marinating time

Cooking time:
5 minutes

*This kebab recipe is quick and easy. Serve the kebabs in a toasted pitta bread pocket for a tasty meal. Alternatively, try them on a bed of rice for a low-potassium, low-fat, protein-rich meal which is also great for people who are on a fluid restriction.*

## Ingredients *(serves 2)*
chicken breasts • 2 medium (about 260 g total)
plain yoghurt • half a small pot (75 g)
green pepper • ½ large
garlic • 1 clove, crushed
onion • ½ medium
mango chutney • 2 teaspoons
curry powder • 2 teaspoons
pitta bread • 2, lightly toasted

You will need four metal kebab skewers.

Crush the garlic and add it to the yoghurt along with the curry powder and mango chutney; mix well.

Cut the chicken into large chunks, add to the marinade and mix well. Leave in the fridge to marinate for at least 1 hour. Meanwhile cut the onion and green pepper into large pieces.

Place alternate pieces of the marinated chicken, pepper and onion on to each of the 4 skewers.

Preheat the grill to medium-high and grill the kebabs for 5 minutes turning frequently. Serve with the pitta breads.

**High protein**
✳
**Low potassium**
✳
**Low phosphate**

## Cook's tip
Use more or less curry powder depending upon how spicy you like your food.

**MEAT AND POULTRY**

# VEGETARIAN MAIN DISHES

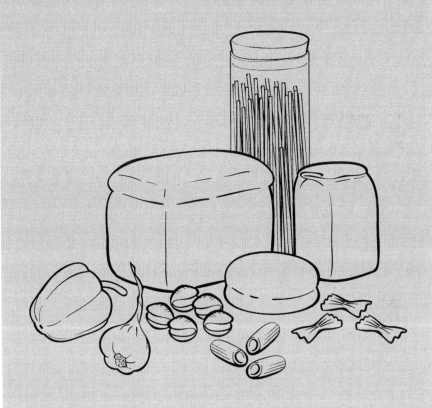

# Carrot, leek and goats' cheese tarts

**Preparation time:**
25 minutes

**Cooking time:**
30 minutes

*These colourful tarts, using ready-made pastry, are a quick and easy vegetarian dish suitable for an informal weekday supper. They also make a great vegetarian starter or main course for a dinner party. Any leftovers taste equally good served cold the next day, and are suitable for taking out as a packed lunch.*

**Ingredients** *(serves 4 as main course, 8 as a starter)*
carrots • 2 medium, peeled and finely sliced
leeks • 2 medium, trimmed and finely sliced
garlic • 1 clove, crushed
olive oil • 1 tablespoon
herbs, e.g. oregano, sage, mixed • 2 teaspoons dried,
   or 2 tablespoons fresh
ready-rolled puff pastry • 375 g pack
soft goats' cheese • 150 g

Preheat the oven to 200°C, Gas Mark 6.
   In a large saucepan, boil the carrots in plenty of water for 5 minutes. Add the leeks and boil for a further 5 minutes. Drain the carrots and leeks well, then return to the pan. Stir in the olive oil, garlic and herbs and leave to cool.
   Cut the pastry into eight squares and place on a baking sheet, lined with baking parchment. Divide the vegetable mixture into eight and spread each pastry square with the mixture, leaving a ½ cm border round the edge. Dot the goat's cheese over the top of the vegetables. Bake for about 30 minutes or until the pastry is golden brown.

High protein
∗
High energy
∗
Low potassium
∗
Low phosphate

### Serving suggestion
These tarts are best served warm rather than piping hot. A boiled green vegetable such as broccoli or green beans, makes a good accompaniment, depending on your vegetable allowance. Another alternative is a green salad. For a more substantial meal, add bread or boiled new potatoes.

# Cauliflower and chickpea curry

*A quick and easy vegetarian curry that does not include tomatoes and uses lower potassium ingredients to keep the potassium content of the dish down. The emphasis is on the traditional Indian spices, rather than salt to keep the sodium content low in this tasty dish.*

**Ingredients** *(serves 4)*
cauliflower • 225 g, divided into small florets
vegetable oil • 1 tablespoon
onion • 1 small, finely chopped
garlic • 1 clove
red lentils • 55 g
garam masala • 2 heaped teaspoons
tinned chickpeas • 450 g can, drained
mango chutney • 2 tablespoons
lemon juice • 1 tablespoon
coriander leaves • fresh, chopped, 1 tablespoon
white rice • 220 g

Boil the cauliflower florets in a large pan of water for 5 minutes or until tender. Drain and reserve.

Meanwhile, heat the oil in a large pan and fry the onion over a medium heat until softened. Stir in the garlic, lentils and garam masala and add 500 ml water. Bring to the boil and simmer for 20 minutes or until the lentils are tender. Meanwhile, boil the rice in unsalted water.

Add the boiled cauliflower, chickpeas, mango chutney and lemon juice to the curry mixture and cook for 5 minutes or until heated through. Garnish with the fresh coriander leaves. Serve with the rice, or with pitta bread, chappattis or other bread.

*Hint*

**High protein**
*
**Low potassium**
*
**Low phosphate**

Boiling the cauliflower separately for a short time helps reduce the potassium content of this dish without affecting its taste. This works well with many other vegetables such as carrots, beans, peas, pumpkin, potatoes, etc.

VEGETARIAN MAIN DISHES

# Cauliflower cheese with red peppers

Preparation time:
15 minutes

Cooking time:
10 minutes

*This is really a cheat's cauliflower cheese as it is so easy but it has the extra advantage in that it is lower in phosphate than the standard version. There is no white sauce to make – crème fraîche works well instead. The boiled cauliflower and red pepper are fairly low in potassium so the dish also works well as a lower potassium vegetarian option.*

**Ingredients** *(serves 2)*
medium cauliflower • 1 (about 225 g)
red pepper • 1 medium
crème fraîche • 200 ml
wholegrain mustard • 1 teaspoon
mature cheddar cheese • 60 g, grated

Preheat the grill to high. Cut the red pepper lengthways into quarters and place on a baking tray, skin-side up. Grill until the skin is blackened, then immediately place the peppers into a small plastic bag. Leave to cool, then peel off the skin and slice up the flesh.

Meanwhile, divide the cauliflower into medium florets. Boil in plenty of water for about 5–8 minutes or until tender, then drain well and place in a shallow ovenproof dish.

Mix together the crème fraîche, mustard, the pepper slices and most of the cheese, reserving about 2 tablespoons of the cheese. Spread the crème fraîche mixture over the cauliflower and then sprinkle with the reserved cheese.

High energy
✳
High protein
✳
Low potassium
✳
Low phosphate

Grill under a medium grill until the top is golden brown. Serve with crusty bread or try with garlic toast (see page 88).

*Hint*
Use half fat crème fraîche to reduce the fat and calorie content of this dish.

# Stir-fried noodles with tofu and mixed vegetables

Preparation time:
15 minutes

Cooking time:
20 minutes

*This is a colourful and tasty vegetarian dish which is easy to adapt for one or for a family supper. It's a good choice if you are on dialysis as it is low in fluid and suitable for those on potassium or phosphate restrictions. Noodles are low in potassium and very quick to prepare and the tofu is a versatile ingredient that can be bought in most supermarkets and provides high-quality protein.*

**Ingredients** *(serves 2)*
dried Chinese egg noodles • 130 g
carrots • 100 g
leeks • 100 g
frozen green beans • 50 g
red pepper • 50 g
sunflower oil • 2 tablespoons
plain firm tofu • 250 g
garlic • 1 clove
Chinese five spice powder • 1 teaspoon
red chilli powder • ½ teaspoon
low-sodium soy sauce • 1 tablespoon
rice wine (or white wine) vinegar • 2 tablespoons
fresh coriander • 2 tablespoons, chopped
freshly ground black pepper • to taste

Cook the noodles according to the packet instructions, drain and leave to cool. Cut the carrots and leeks into thin slices and boil with the green beans in plenty of unsalted water for 5 minutes. Then drain well. Finely slice the red pepper. Drain the tofu and cut into bite-size cubes.

Heat the oil in a large non-stick wok or frying pan over a medium-high heat. Add the tofu and stir fry for 5–8 minutes until lightly browned. Remove from the pan and set aside. Heat the remainder of the oil and add the vegetables in the following order, stir-frying briefly between each addition: carrots, leeks, green beans, red peppers, garlic. Then stir in the five spice and chilli powder followed by the tofu. Then add the cooked noodles and allow to heat through for 1–2 minutes.

High protein
✳
Low potassium
✳
Low phosphate

**VEGETARIAN MAIN DISHES**

Just before serving mix in the soy sauce, vinegar, fresh coriander and black pepper. Serve immediately.

**Cook's tip 1:** At the table you could serve some finely sliced spring onions, lightly toasted sesame seeds and cashew nuts for those who are not restricting their phosphate or potassium intakes.

**Cook's tip 2:** For those who are missing a savoury nutty taste, try a sprinkle of sesame seed oil on noodles, couscous or bulgar wheat, or on vegetables such as boiled carrots, cauliflower or green beans.

# *Tabuleh*

*Tabuleh uses bulgar wheat which is a great low-potassium, starchy alternative to potatoes. This dish works well as a hot main meal or cold as a salad in the summer. A variation of the dish can also be made using rice or couscous.*

**Ingredients** *(serves 2)*
bulgar wheat • 120 g
cucumber • 50 g, finely diced
red pepper • half, finely diced
fresh coriander • 2 tablespoons, finely chopped
fresh mint • 2 tablespoons, finely chopped
   (or 2 teaspoons concentrated mint sauce)
lemon • 1, juice only
olive oil • 1 tablespoon
spring onions • 2, finely chopped
red kidney beans • 1 tin (400 g), drained
pepper • to taste

To rehydrate the bulgar wheat, follow the packet instructions or try the following speedy method. Place in a microwavable dish and pour over boiling water to just above the surface of the wheat. Microwave for 2 minutes and leave to stand for 10 minutes, then drain away any excess water and leave to cool to room temperature.

Add all of the remaining ingredients to the bulgar wheat. Stir well and season with pepper to taste.

**High protein**
✳
**Low potassium**
✳
**Low phosphate**

**Cook's tip:** Chopped cooked meat or tinned fish (for non-vegetarians) or additional vegetables could be added instead of the beans, depending on your preferences and dietary needs.

# Tricolore pasta

*We are always being asked for suggestions for 'no tomato' pasta recipes by people on low-potassium diets. This recipe works well for people who eat pasta regularly and want an alternative dish that looks as good as it tastes.*

**Ingredients** *(serves 2)*
pasta shapes (twists, shells, bows) • 120 g
fresh parsley • 2 tablespoons, chopped
red chilli • half (or more, to taste) deseeded
    and finely diced
garlic • 3 cloves, crushed
olive oil • 2 tablespoons
cheddar cheese • 20 g, grated, to garnish (optional)

Boil the pasta for about 10 minutes or according to the instructions on the packet. Drain in a strainer or colander.

Low potassium
＊
Low phosphate

While the pasta is draining, toss the parsley, chilli and garlic together in the still warm pasta pan with the olive oil, and heat gently for about half a minute. Add this mixture to the drained pasta and garnish with some grated cheese.

# Vegetable frittata

*This is an extra-special omelette, ideal as a quick lunch or supper for two, but easily adapted for four or more just by increasing the amounts of all the ingredients. The recipe uses mainly egg whites so it is a great low-phosphate, high-protein, vegetarian option suitable for the whole family.*

**Ingredients** *(serves 2)*
fresh or frozen peas • 50 g
cooking oil • 2 teaspoons
onion • 1 small (50 g), finely chopped
egg • 2 whole eggs and whites of 2 more
red pepper • 50 g
fresh herbs (e.g.parsley, chives, basil) • 1 tablespoon, finely chopped
freshly ground black pepper • to taste
cheddar, grated • 20 g (optional)

You will need a small, non-stick, frying pan.

Boil the peas in plenty of water, then remove from the heat and drain. Preheat the grill to medium-high.

In a separate bowl, beat the egg and egg whites together with the herbs and a pinch of black pepper. Over a medium heat, soften the onion and pepper in the oil and stir in the peas. Pour the egg mixture into the pan and cook without stirring for 2–3 minutes, lifting up the edge of the omelette with a spatula so the uncooked egg can flow underneath.

If you are using grated cheese, sprinkle it onto the top. Place the frying pan under the grill and cook for 3–4 minutes until the frittata is just set and the cheese is beginning to brown. (But be careful with the pan handle if it is not heat resistant.)

Serve immediately, with bread or new potatoes.

High protein
✳
Low potassium
✳
Low phosphate

**Cook's tip 1:** You can adapt this recipe in order to use up leftover boiled vegetables.

**Cook's tip 2:** Use the same idea of mixing whole egg with additional egg whites to make scrambled egg or a standard omelette.

# SIDE DISHES

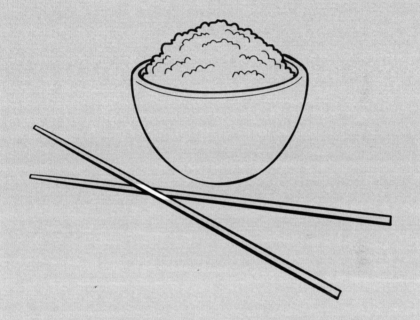

# Golden spiced couscous

**Preparation time:**
10 minutes

**Cooking time:**
10 minutes

*Couscous is a North African staple and makes a great low-potassium alternative to other starchy accompaniments such as potatoes, yam, plantain or breadfruit. It is very quick to prepare and this recipe uses spices and herbs for flavouring instead of salt. Try the golden couscous with curry, stews, plain roast meat or fish dishes. It is good if you are having sausages, burgers or other processed meat products as its low sodium content will go some way towards compensating for the saltiness of the other foods.*

**Ingredients** *(serves 4)*
sunflower oil • 1 tablespoon
onion • 1 small, finely chopped
ground turmeric • ½ teaspoon
ground cumin • 1 teaspoon
couscous • 225 g
boiling water • 600 ml
black pepper • freshly ground, to taste
fresh coriander or parsley • 1 tablespoon, chopped

You will need a large saucepan with tightly fitting lid. Heat the oil in a large saucepan over a medium heat. Add the onion and cook for 3–4 minutes until softened. Stir in the turmeric and cumin and cook for 1 minute. Stir in the couscous. Add the boiling water. Stir briefly, remove from the heat, cover and leave to stand for approx 5 minutes.

Fluff up with a fork. Stir in the pepper and fresh herbs immediately before serving.

**Low potassium**

\*

**Low phosphate**

**Cook's tip:** Try adding 300 g mixed frozen vegetables, boiled according to packet instructions, to the couscous with the herbs and black pepper. Don't forget to include this in your vegetable allowance if you are on a potassium restriction.

# Golden spiced couscous (cont'd)

### More suggestions

This dish can be served cold as a salad with or without the added vegetables or other vegetables to suit. If you like the taste, mix in a little homemade French dressing or just drizzle with salad oil and lemon or vinegar. The couscous salad is great for a buffet or summer barbecue.

For a really easy packed lunch stir in some tinned tuna, chopped boiled eggs, diced cold meat or drained tinned chickpeas or other beans, depending on your dietary allowances and personal preferences.

SIDE DISHES

# Mashed potato with a difference

**Preparation time:**
15 minutes

**Cooking time:**
15 minutes

*Most people on a low-potassium diet are advised to boil their potatoes to reduce the potassium content, making mash an ideal choice. We have added a few tasty ingredients to the standard recipe to help make this a bit more interesting. Using olive oil instead of the traditional butter is a healthy way to make your mashed potato creamy and delicious with or without the extra flavours.*

### Ingredients *(serves 2)*
potatoes • 300 g, boiled and water discarded
olive oil • 1 tablespoon

### Options

#### Cheesy mash
red Leicester cheese • 40 g, grated
Dijon mustard • 1 teaspoon

#### Mustard mash
Dijon mustard • 2 teaspoon
wholegrain mustard • 2 teaspoons

CHEESY MASH
High energy
✳
High protein
✳
Low phosphate

#### Garlic and herb mash
garlic • 2 cloves, crushed
fresh parsley and/or chives • 1 tablespoon, chopped

For all the options above except the garlic and herb mixture, simply combine all the ingredients together and mash well. You can warm the mixture back up to serving temperature if it has cooled by heating it in the microwave for 30–60 seconds.

MUSTARD MASH
and
GARLIC
AND HERB MASH
✳
Low phosphate

For the garlic and herb mixture, to avoid too harsh a taste, microwave the garlic in the tablespoon of olive oil for 30 seconds (or heat in a small pan until softened). Add this to the potato with the chopped herbs, and mash well.

# Thai fragrant rice

**Preparation time:**
5 minutes

**Cooking time:**
20 minutes

*This is a tasty spin on plain boiled rice. The bonus is that it that rice is naturally a low-fat, low-phosphate, low-potassium food and cooked this way needs no salt. It has quite a subtle taste so it is best served with milder dishes.*

**Ingredients** *(serves 2)*
plain white rice • 110 g
lemon grass • 1 stick, gashed several times
coriander seeds • 2 teaspoons

Make your rice in the usual way, but add the lemon grass and coriander seeds to the boiling water.

Once the rice is cooked remove the lemon grass stick and serve.

### Cook's tip
Boiled brown rice is another good low-potassium alternative to potatoes. It is high in fibre and has a delicious nutty taste. It can be served hot (mix in some butter or margarine to increase the calorie content) or try it as a base for a cold salad mixed with a little French dressing and chopped chives or diced onion.

Low potassium
*
Low phosphate

SIDE DISHES

# DESSERTS

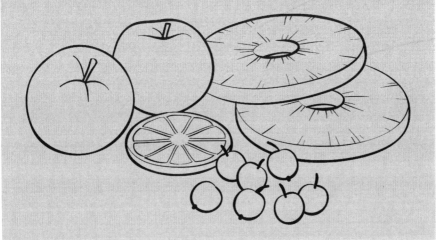

# Apple and cinnamon oat crumble

**Preparation time:**
20 minutes

**Cooking time:**
40–50 minutes

*This is a traditional dessert with a hint of spice. Apples are a lower potassium fruit and oats add a crunchy taste which is high in soluble fibre. If you are on a low-potassium diet, count one portion of crumble as one fruit portion.*

## Ingredients *(serves 4)*
cooking apples • 450 g peeled, cored and thinly sliced
brown sugar • 75 g
plain flour • 100 g
rolled oats • 75 g
ground cinnamon • 2 teaspoons
butter or (hard) margarine • 75 g

Preheat the oven to 190°C /Gas Mark 5.
    Place the sliced apple in a small ovenproof pie dish and sprinkle with 25 g (1 oz) of the sugar.
    Mix the flour, oats, cinnamon and remaining sugar together in a bowl. Cut up the butter or margarine into small pieces. Add to the oats and rub in with your fingers until the mixture is crumbly.
    Sprinkle the crumble mixture evenly over the fruit. Bake for 40–50 minutes, until the crumble is golden brown and the fruit juices are bubbling up the side of the dish.
    Serve with whipped cream or crème fraîche.

### For a change
High energy
※
High protein
※
Low potassium
※
Low phosphate

Try making this recipe using pears instead of apples and adding 1 teaspoon ginger instead of cinnamon to the crumble mixture

### Hint
Cream and crème fraîche are lower in potassium and phosphate than ice cream or custard.

# Cinnamon rice pudding

**Preparation time:**
15 minutes

**Cooking time:**
1 ½ hours

*This is a version of a traditional comfort food. As with all rice pudding recipes, it can take a while to cook but it's worth it. In this recipe the potassium and phosphate content has been reduced by replacing some of the milk with double cream and water. If you are diabetic you could also substitute sweetener for the sugar.*

**Ingredients** *(serves 4)*
pudding rice • 100 g
whole milk • 280 ml (½ pint)
double cream • 280ml (½ pint)
water • 280ml (½ pint)
sugar • 80 g
vanilla essence • 1 teaspoon
cinnamon • 1 teaspoon (or to taste)

**High energy**
✳
**High protein**
✳
**Low potassium**
✳
**Low phosphate**
✳
**Suitable for diabetics**
**(if using sweetener)**

Put all the ingredients except the vanilla and cinnamon into a pan and stir well. Heat at a medium to low heat setting, stirring regularly for about 1 hour.
　　Once the rice is cooked stir in the vanilla essence and add cinnamon to taste, warming through for about another 10 minutes.

*Cook's tip*
Instead of cinnamon, try adding nutmeg, or garnish with a little jam or apple purée.

# Cranachan

**Preparation time:**
20 minutes

**Cooking time:**
1–2 hours

*This is a traditional Scottish dessert that is similar to a trifle but much simpler to make. It is high in energy (calories) but lower in potassium and phosphate as it doesn't contain milk. The raspberries (or strawberries) in one portion of cranachan will count as one fruit portion if you are on a potassium restriction.*

**Ingredients** *(serves 4)*
clear honey • 4 tablespoons
whisky • 45 ml (3 tablespoons)
rolled oats • 55 g
double cream • 300 ml
raspberries (or strawberries) • 340 g

Warm the honey with the whisky in a small pan, remove from the heat and leave to cool.

Meanwhile spread the oats out on a baking tray in a thin layer and place under a medium grill. Toast, stirring occasionally, until browned. Leave to cool.

Whip the cream in a large bowl until stiff, taking care not to over-whip. Gently stir in the oats, honey and whisky.

Reserving four whole raspberries for decoration, stir the remaining raspberries into the cream mixture. Divide between four glass dishes and top with the reserved raspberries. Cover and chill for 1–2 hours before serving.

**Cook's tip:** Scottish raspberries are delicious but are often difficult to find out of season. If you can't find fresh raspberries try using the same weight of frozen or tinned (drained) raspberries or even strawberries for this recipe. Tinned raspberries have the advantage of containing about half the potassium of fresh raspberries of the same weight.

**High energy**
✳
**Low potassium**
✳
**Low phosphate**
✳
**Suitable for diabetics**
**(see tip)**

**If you have diabetes:** Omit the honey. Toast the oats as above, place in a bowl and sprinkle with the whisky (no need to heat through). Add the oats and raspberries to the cream as above and sweeten to taste with a granulated artificial sweetener.

# Lemon and blueberry creams

**Preparation time:**
15 minutes

**Cooking time:**
30 minutes

**Chilling time:**
1 hour minimum
24–26 hours
maximum

*This is a truly indulgent dessert that is very easy to make. It would be perfect for a romantic meal for two or a cosy meal for one (save the other portion for next day). On the other hand you could scale the quantities of ingredients up to cater for a large dinner party or buffet, especially as it can be made the day before. The creams contain protein and are high in energy, making this an ideal dish to have after or between your meals if your appetite is poor. The fruity flavour may appeal if you are suffering from taste changes.*

**Ingredients** *(makes 2 portions)*
blueberries • 30 g
double cream • 200 ml
lemon curd • 60 g
egg whites • 2
caster sugar • 1 tablespoon

You will also need 2 small ramekin dishes.

Preheat the oven to 150°C, Gas Mark 2.

Divide the blueberries between the ramekin dishes. In a small pan, heat the cream gently until it bubbles round the edge and stir in the lemon curd. Meanwhile, add the sugar to the egg white in a mixing bowl and whisk until well mixed.

Gradually whisk in the cream mixture. Divide the mixture between the two ramekins. Place the ramekins in a shallow roasting container, filled with boiling water to a depth of 2–3 cm. Bake in the oven for 25–30 minutes or until the custard is set. Remove and cool. Chill for a minimum of 1 hour or overnight. Serve alone or with any light and crispy biscuit, such as tuiles, ginger thins, rich tea fingers etc.

**High energy**
✳
**High protein**
✳
**Low potassium**
✳
**Low phosphate**

**Cook's tip:** Many other fruits work well with this recipe. If you are on a reduced potassium diet check which fruits fit in with your allowances. Tinned fruits and fresh berries and defrosted frozen berries can be used without prior cooking. Other fresh fruits such as peaches, pears or cherries will need to be softened by cooking first.

# Lemon surprise pudding

**Preparation time:**
20 minutes

**Cooking time:**
35 minutes

*The 'surprise' in this pudding is the layer of lemon sauce, which forms below the sponge as it cooks. This makes it good for fluid-restricted diets as no extra sauce is needed.*

**Ingredients** *(serves 4)*
low-salt butter or soft margarine • 50 g
milk • 150 ml
plain flour • 50 g
lemon • 1, grated rind and juice
eggs • 2, separated
caster sugar • 100 g

You will also need a 600 ml/l pint ovenproof dish, and a roasting tin large enough to hold this dish. Preheat the oven to 190°C (Gas Mark 5).

Lightly grease the ovenproof dish. Cream the butter or margarine with the sugar. Then beat in the milk, flour, lemon rind, juice and egg yolks. Whisk the egg whites until they form stiff peaks and fold into the lemon mixture, using a metal spoon.

Pour the mixture into the greased dish. Stand this dish in a roasting tin and pour water into the tin to a depth of 2–3 cm. Bake for about 35 minutes or until golden brown. Serve the pudding immediately.

**High energy**
∗
**High protein**
∗
**Low potassium**
∗
**Low phosphate**

# Mandarin cheesecake

**Preparation time:**
30 minutes

**Chilling time:**
50 minutes

*This is an old favourite which works as well for a dinner party as for an everyday dessert. If you are preparing the cheesecake ahead, the mixture can be made the day before, but keep the biscuit base crunchy by mixing it on the day that it is needed.*

**Ingredients** *(serves 6)*
low-salt butter or margarine • 50 g
digestive biscuits • 100 g, crushed
curd or cream cheese • 250 g
caster sugar • 50 g
   (or equivalent of suitable sweetener)
orange • 1, grated rind and juice
double cream • 170 mls, whipped
mandarin oranges • 1 small tin, for decoration
fresh mint • 4 leaves (optional)

**High energy**
✳
**Low potassium**
✳
**Low phosphate**
✳
**Suitable for diabetics**
**(if using sweetener)**

Melt the margarine and stir in the crushed biscuits. Press the mixture onto a base of a quiche dish and leave in the fridge for 20 minutes or until firm.

Mix the curd cheese with the sugar, orange rind, juice and whipped cream. Spoon the mixture onto the biscuit base and leave in the fridge for another 30 minutes.

Before serving, decorate the topping with the mandarin oranges and mint.

# Pears in white wine

**Preparation time:**
10 minutes

**Cooking time:**
30 minutes (including
standing time)

*This is an easy dessert for a special occasion. White wine is lower in potassium than red, and you can omit the mascarpone for those on a low-fat diet. If you use artificial sweetener, do check first that it is a type suitable for cooking.*

*Any pears left over can be kept in the fridge and served chilled within 24 hours.*

### Ingredients *(serves 4)*
small pears • 4 (not too soft)
white wine • 250 ml
cloves • about 8
cinnamon stick • 1 (optional)
orange • 1 (zest only)
sugar • 1 tablespoon (or granulated sweetener)
mascarpone • 100 g
brown sugar/artificial granulated sweetener to serve

Peel and core the pears. Cut in half lengthways and place in a saucepan. Pour over the white wine. Add the cloves, cinnamon stick (if using), and the sugar or sweetener.

Remove the peel from the orange with a vegetable peeler, trying not to remove too much of the white pith, and add to the pan. Heat gently, until just bubbling. Lower heat, cover pan and simmer gently until pears are tender, (about 10–15 minutes).

Remove pan from the heat and leave to stand for a further 15 minutes. Remove pears from the pan with a slotted spoon. Discard the wine and spice mixture. Serve while still warm on individual plates, with a spoonful of mascarpone on the side. Sprinkle with brown sugar or artificial sweetener to taste.

**High energy**
✻
**Low potassium**
✻
**Low phosphate**
✻
**Suitable for diabetics**
**(if using sweetener)**

### Cook's tip
Use low-fat yoghurt, cream or ice cream instead of mascarpone, depending on your dietary restrictions and preferences.

# Pineapple with rum and ginger

Preparation time:
10–15 minutes

Cooking time:
7 minutes

*Pineapple can make a good dessert or snack all by itself. Adding a few Caribbean inspired ingredients makes it a little naughtier but very nice! This quick and easy dessert can be made with either fresh or tinned pineapple. It would be equally delicious whether you are cooking for just one or for a whole group of people. Just make more or less, as required. If you can't find preserved ginger try using some ginger marmalade or powdered ginger instead.*

**Ingredients** *(serves 2)*
fresh pineapple • 200 g (skin and core removed)
butter or margarine • 10 g
preserved ginger in syrup • 1 tablespoon (20 g)
    chopped, plus 2 teaspoons of the syrup
brown sugar • 1 tablespoon
rum • 2 tablespoons

Slice the pineapple and cut into chunks. Heat the butter or margarine in a non-stick wok or frying pan. Add the pineapple and cook over a medium heat for a minute or two. Add the ginger, syrup and brown sugar and cook for a further 5 minutes.

Sprinkle the rum over the mixture and remove from the heat. Serve immediately with some good quality ice cream (vanilla and toffee/maple syrup flavours work well) or cream or mascarpone mixed with a drop of vanilla essence per serving. For a lower fat dessert use low-fat plain yoghurt instead.

**For a change:** Try making this recipe using fresh apples with powdered cinnamon instead of ginger and brandy instead of rum.

**Hint:** 100 g fresh pineapple contains a modest 4 mmol potassium. The same weight of tinned pineapple contains just under half this, making it a great choice for a low-potassium diet.

Low potassium
✳
Low phosphate
✳
Suitable for diabetics
(if using sweetener)

**For diabetics and healthy eating fans:** Use powdered spices and add a granulated sweetener instead of the sugar and syrup to keep the sugar content down.

# EASY BAKING

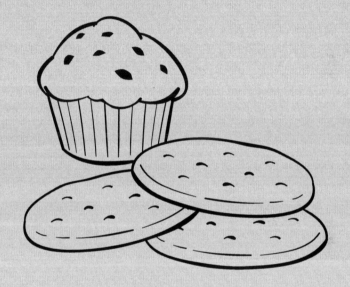

# 'Bakewell' muffins

**Preparation time:**
20 minutes

**Cooking time:**
15–20 minutes

*American muffins are simple to make and this version will remind you of Bakewell tart. Almond essence is a great way to add a flavour of almonds without the nuts themselves, which you may be avoiding if you are on a low-potassium or low-phosphate diet.*

**Ingredients** *(makes about 12)*
self-raising flour • 270 g
granulated sugar • 185 g
milk • 250 ml
eggs • 2, lightly beaten
sunflower, corn or rapeseed oil • 150 ml
almond essence • 1–2 teaspoons
raspberry jam • approx 100 g

You will need a muffin tin, lined with paper cases. Preheat the oven to 220°C, Gas Mark 7.

In a large bowl combine the flour and sugar. Make a well in the centre. In a separate bowl or jug combine the milk, oil, eggs and almond essence and then add this mixture to the dry ingredients. Very lightly mix together until all the ingredients are only just combined. Be very careful not to overmix – the mixture should look like a very lumpy batter.

Spoon the mixture into the muffin cases – they should be about three-quarters full. Top each with a teaspoon of raspberry jam. Bake in the pre-heated oven for about 15–20 minutes or until well risen and lightly browned. The jam should sink down into the middle of the muffin while it is cooking.

Remove muffins from the tin and leave to cool on a wire rack. The muffins keep for 3–4 days in an airtight container.

**High energy**
✳
**Low potassium**
✳
**Low phosphate**

### Cook's tip

For a chocolate 'fix', try topping each muffin with 4 or 5 plain chocolate drops instead of the jam. If you are on a low-potassium or low-phosphate diet, you may have been advised not to eat chocolate. However, this will add minimal amounts of phosphate and potassium to this recipe (0.1 ml phosphate, 0.2 ml potassium per muffin). Our tasters have found that this hint of chocolate works really well with the almondy taste of the muffin.

# Breakfast muffins

**Preparation time:**
30 minutes
plus approx
65 minutes rising time

*Although these do need to include a little salt, they are much lower in sodium than shop-bought muffins, crumpets or rolls. They are great served with poached eggs, cottage cheese or a little butter and jam at any time of day*

**Cooking time:**
5–14 minutes,
depending on pan size

### Ingredients *(for 6 muffins)*
full fat milk • 115 ml, hand hot
salt • 1 pinch
water • 1 tablespoon
easy blend yeast • 6 g (approx 2 level teaspoons)
plain flour • 225 g

Sift the flour and salt into a bowl. Make a well in the centre and mix in the liquid to form a soft dough. If it is a little sticky add some more flour, or water if it is a little dry.

Knead the dough for 10 minutes, then return it to the bowl. Cover and leave to prove in a warm place for around 40 minutes.

Roll the dough out to 2–3 cm thick, and cut into rounds of approximately 7 cm. Place on baking tray, cover and leave to rise again this time for around 25 minutes.

Cook the muffins on a low heat in a heavy pan, or on a griddle rubbed with a bit of butter or margarine. They should require 5–7 minutes on each side.

### Hint
Use wholemeal flour to increase the fibre content of the muffins. You may need to add 1–2 teaspoons more water when mixing the dough.

High protein
✳
Low potassium
✳
Low phosphate

### Cook's tip
Try adding 1–2 teaspoons of cinnamon powder to the flour before sifting.

# Butterscotch shortbread

**Preparation time:**
10 minutes

**Cooking time:**
35 minutes

*This makes a light biscuit with a fudgy taste which is quick and easy to make and a delicious twist on the traditional recipe.*

**Ingredients** *(makes 8 slices)*
low-salt butter or margarine • 110 g (softened)
dark brown sugar • 55 g
vanilla essence • ½ teaspoon
plain flour • 155 g
caster sugar • 1 tablespoon (optional)

Preheat the oven to 160°C (Gas Mark 3).

Cream the sugar and fat together until light and fluffy. Stir in the vanilla essence. Mix in the flour. Knead the mixture together until it forms a firm dough. Turn out on to a floured surface and roll or press out into a round shape, approximately 1½ cm. Place onto a lightly greased baking tray and prick all over with a fork. Bake for about 35–40 minutes.

Sprinkle with caster sugar (if using) and cut into eight pieces while still hot. Leave to cool before eating.

The shortbread can be stored in an airtight container for several days.

**High energy**
✳
**Low potassium**
✳
**Low phosphate**

# Florida fruit cake

**Preparation time:**
20 minutes

**Cooking time:**
60–70 minutes

*This light cake is simple and quick to make and has a subtle taste of oranges. It is a great alternative to dried fruit cake, especially if you are on a low-potassium diet. As only one egg is used, it is also lower in phosphate than many other sponge cakes.*

**Ingredients** *(makes 10 slices)*
self raising flour • 225 g
low-salt butter or hard margarine • 100 g
   (cold from the fridge)
sugar • 100 g
candied mixed peel • 100 g
egg • 1 beaten
fresh orange juice • 30 ml (2 tablespoons)
milk • approx 90 ml (6 tablespoons)

You will need a 700 g (1½ lb) loaf tin.

Preheat the oven to 180°C (Gas Mark 4). Grease the loaf tin and line the base and the longer sides with a single rectangle of baking parchment. Put the flour into a large bowl and rub in the butter until the mixture looks like fine breadcrumbs. Stir in the sugar and the mixed peel. Then, with a metal spoon, gradually mix in the egg, orange juice and milk. If you hold a spoon of mixture above the bowl, the mixture should drop back into the bowl by the time you count slowly to five. If it does not, add 1–2 tablespoons more milk.

Pour the mixture into the tin and smooth over the top. Bake for about 60–70 minutes, until light golden brown and firm to the touch. Cool in the tin for about 5 minutes and then turn out onto a wire rack to cool.

***Cook's tip:***
To store for 3–4 days, wrap the cake tightly in foil when completely cold. For longer storage the cake also freezes well. You could also cut the cake into thick slices before freezing and then just take a slice out at a time, cover with clingfilm and defrost overnight. This is particularly useful if you live alone.

**High energy**
✳
**Low potassium**
✳
**Low phosphate**

# Ginger and cherry flapjacks

**Preparation time:**
10 minutes

**Cooking time:**
20 minutes

*These are quick and simple to make and are a great high-calorie snack to eat between meals. Glacé cherries are a low-potassium treat and can be used instead of dried fruit in homemade biscuits and cakes. If you don't like glacé cherries, just leave them out or use some candied mixed peel instead.*

**Ingredients** *(makes about 10)*
low-salt butter or margarine • 85 g
sugar • 55 g
honey • 2 tablespoons (approx 80 g)
glacé cherries • 55 g, chopped
ground ginger • 1 teaspoon
porridge oats • 200 g

Lightly grease a small baking tin (approx 15 cm × 20 cm). Melt the fat in a large pan over a low heat, and stir in the sugar and honey. Add the cherries and ground ginger and stir in the oats, making sure they are well coated.

**High energy**
✲
**Low potassium**
✲
**Low phosphate**

Press the mixture into the baking tin and bake for approximately 20 minutes at 180°C (Gas Mark 4). Cut into squares while still warm and leave to cool before eating. Store in an airtight container when cold.

# Appendix 1
# Useful addresses and websites

**National Kidney Federation**
6 Stanley Street
Worksop
Nottinghamshire
S81 7HX
Tel: 01909 487795
Fax: 01909 481723
Helpline: 0845 601 02 09
Website: www.kidney.org.uk

**Kidney Research UK**
King's Chambers
Priestgate
Peterborough
PE1 1FG
Tel: 0845 070 7601
Helpline: 0845 300 14 99
Email: info@kidneyresearchuk.org
Website: www.kidneyresearchuk.org

**Diabetes UK**
10 Parkway
London
NW1 7AA
Tel: 020 7424 1000
Fax: 020 7424 1001
Helpline: 0845 120 29 60
Website: www.diabetes.org.uk

**The British Dietetic Association**
5th Floor
Charles House
148–9 Great Charles Street
Queensway
Birmingham
B3 3HT
Tel 0121 200 8080
Fax 0121 200 8081
Website: www.bda.uk.com

# Appendix 2 – Nutritional analysis of recipes per portion

| Recipe | Protein (g) | Energy (kcals) | Potassium (mg) | Phosphorous (mg) | Sodium (mg) | Sodium/ 100 g food |
|---|---|---|---|---|---|---|
| Apple and cinnamon oat crumble | 5 | 407 | 245 | 113 | 21 | 11 |
| 'Bakewell' muffins | 4 | 297 | 83 | 141 | 106 | 119 |
| Beef and mushroom stroganoff | 34 | 652 | 654 | 379 | 325 | 98 |
| Breakfast muffins | 5 | 142 | 106 | 72 | 75 | 123 |
| Butterscotch shortbread | 2 | 203 | 43 | 25 | 7 | 16 |
| Carnival chicken with peppers and rice | 27 | 538 | 790 | 214 | 142 | 27 |
| Carrot, leek and goats' cheese tarts | 15 | 526 | 311 | 174 | 546 | 205 |
| Cauliflower and chickpea curry | 15 | 417 | 548 | 231 | 367 | 160 |
| Cauliflower cheese with red peppers | 15 | 570 | 382 | 300 | 360 | 109 |
| Cheesy cheat's pizza | 16 | 269 | 438 | 284 | 571 | 272 |
| Cheesy mashed potato | 8 | 241 | 442 | 146 | 211 | 118 |
| Chicken and mushroom pastry parcels | 23 | 823 | 417 | 241 | 428 | 159 |
| Chicken with capers | 34 | 477 | 836 | 391 | 423 | 111 |
| Chilli burgers with relishes | 21 | 306 | 420 | 263 | 424 | 231 |
| Cinnamon rice pudding | 5 | 563 | 186 | 127 | 48 | 19 |
| Cranachan | 4 | 560 | 260 | 123 | 27 | 13 |
| Crispy tangy fish | 34 | 383 | 636 | 415 | 417 | 154 |
| Crunchy olive and lime plaice | 24 | 252 | 479 | 278 | 464 | 251 |
| Felafel | 15 | 352 | 438 | 238 | 488 | 200 |
| Fish steaks with orange and mustard | 21 | 251 | 469 | 276 | 168 | 109 |
| Flavoured butters: | | | | | | |
| Chilli and lime | 0 | 63 | 12 | 3 | 3 | 21 |
| Lemon and parsley | 0 | 63 | 24 | 4 | 3 | 25 |

| Item | | | | | | |
|---|---|---|---|---|---|---|
| Florida fruit cake | 3 | 226 | 66 | 125 | 124 | 177 |
| Garlic and herb mashed potato | 3 | 164 | 482 | 58 | 12 | 7 |
| Garlic chicken | 22 | 286 | 548 | 152 | 91 | 39 |
| Ginger and cherry flapjacks | 3 | 203 | 86 | 80 | 12 | 25 |
| Golden spiced couscous | 4 | 158 | 67 | 148 | 3 | 1 |
| Grilled marinated chicken | 31 | 203 | 502 | 291 | 436 | 274 |
| Lamb boulangère | 29 | 430 | 962 | 348 | 102 | 25 |
| Lemon and blueberry creams | 5 | 640 | 129 | 69 | 103 | 55 |
| Lemon surprise pudding | 6 | 299 | 126 | 109 | 61 | 51 |
| Mandarin cheesecake | 3 | 509 | 163 | 80 | 236 | 165 |
| Mustard mashed potato | 4 | 174 | 446 | 70 | 272 | 162 |
| Pears in white wine | 1 | 208 | 251 | 43 | 81 | 47 |
| Pineapple with rum and ginger | 1 | 145 | 179 | 13 | 6 | 5 |
| Pitta crisps with tzatziki | 5 | 158 | 141 | 78 | 226 | 288 |
| Plaice with a creamy coriander topping | 22 | 254 | 453 | 263 | 258 | 151 |
| Pork with a honey and mustard glaze | 28 | 470 | 471 | 269 | 163 | 93 |
| Pork with basil and egg noodles | 31 | 459 | 674 | 385 | 175 | 77 |
| Pork with caramelised apple and crème fraîche | 30 | 650 | 599 | 298 | 93 | 33 |
| Stilton spread with Melba toast | 4 | 223 | 109 | 89 | 237 | 395 |
| Stir-fried noodles, tofu and vegetables | 20 | 491 | 566 | 307 | 517 | 135 |
| Tabuleh | 15 | 405 | 712 | 388 | 478 | 167 |
| Tandoori style kebabs | 43 | 450 | 948 | 478 | 607 | 169 |
| Thai fishcakes | 40 | 535 | 872 | 348 | 407 | 111 |
| Thai fragrant rice | 4 | 199 | 112 | 71 | 5 | 8 |
| Tricolore pasta | 11 | 357 | 276 | 184 | 78 | 78 |
| Tuna pasta Niçoise | 29 | 609 | 479 | 329 | 520 | 203 |
| Tuna pâté | 11 | 116 | 199 | 122 | 260 | 322 |
| Tuna steaks with caramelised shallots | 30 | 205 | 548 | 300 | 62 | 35 |
| Vegetable frittata | 15 | 201 | 288 | 213 | 217 | 120 |

All nutrient analyses in the table on pages 148–9 have been calculated using Dietplan6 with additional data from the USDA website (United States Department of Agriculture – www.usda.gov). They are based on food weight and food selection according to available data, recipe specification or standard food portion sizes as defined in *Food Portion Sizes*, 2nd edition, by the Ministry of Agriculture, Fisheries and Food, 1993. It should be borne in mind that food portions served at home are likely to vary slightly in size, but every effort has been made to be as accurate as possible within this limitation.

The codings categorise recipes by nutrient content and are adapted from British Dietetic Association members' guidelines. They are intended as a general guide only, not as recommendations for any one individual's diet. Suitable choices for each individual will depend on complete daily food selection, medical condition and other factors. Please see your doctor or dietitian for individualised advice.

# Index

*Have you found* **Eating Well with Kidney Failure** *useful and practical? If so, you may be interested in other books from Class Publishing.*

## Kidney Failure Explained     £17.99

*Dr Andy Stein and Janet Wild*

This fully updated new edition of the complete reference manual gives you, your family and friends, the information you really want to know about managing your kidney condition. Written by two experienced medical authors, this practical handbook covers every aspect of living with kidney disease – from diagnosis, drugs and treatment, to diet, relationships and sex.

> 'This book is, without doubt, the best resource currently available for kidney patients and those who care for them.'
> Val Said, kidney transplant patient

## Kidney Dialysis and Transplants – Answers at your fingertips     £14.99

*Dr Andy Stein and Janet Wild with Juliet Auer*

A practical handbook for anyone with long-term kidney failure or their families. The book contains answers to over 450 real questions actually asked by people with end-stage renal failure, and offers positive, clear and medically accurate advice on every aspect of living with the condition.

> 'A first class book on kidney dialysis and transplants that is simple and accurate, and can be used to equal advantage by doctors and their patients.'
> Dr Thomas Stuttaford
> *The Times*

## Kidney Transplants Explained     £17.99

*Dr Andy Stein, Dr Rob Higgins and Janet Wild*

A successful kidney transplant can transform the life of a person with kidney failure, but it is essential to be thoroughly prepared.

   This book answers all your questions about transplants and what they involve. Indispensable to people considering having a transplant or already living with one, it will also be valuable for anyone thinking about donating a kidney.

## Living Well with Kidney Failure     £14.99

*Juliet Auer*

This practical and inspiring book will give you the confidence to live a full and rewarding life. It highlights the experiences of a number of very different people, from all walks of life, ages and family situations. These shared personal accounts celebrate the fullness of life that people living with kidney failure can, and do, achieve.

## Type 1 Diabetes – Answers at your fingertips     £14.99
## Type 2 Diabetes – Answers at your fingertips     £14.99

*both by Dr Charles Fox and Dr Anne Kilvert*

The latest edition of our bestselling reference guide on diabetes has now been split into two books covering the two distinct forms of the disease. These books provide practical advice for patients on every aspect of living with the condition.

# PRIORITY ORDER FORM

*Cut out or photocopy this form and send it (post free in the UK) to:*

**Class Publishing Priority Service**   **Tel: 01256 302 699**
**FREEPOST 16705**       **Fax: 01256 812 558**
**Macmillan Distribution**
**Basingstoke RG21 6ZZ**

**Please send me urgently**       *Post included*
*(tick boxes below)*       *price per copy (UK only)*

☐ **Eating Well with Kidney Failure** (ISBN 9781859591161)  **£17.99**

☐ **Kidney Failure Explained** (ISBN 9781859591451)  **£20.99**

☐ **Kidney Dialysis and Transplants – Answers at your fingertips**  **£17.99**
 (ISBN 9781859590461)

☐ **Kidney Transplants Explained** (ISBN 9781859591932)  **£20.99**

☐ **Living Well with Kidney Failure** (ISBN 9781859591123)  **£17.99**

☐ **Type 1 Diabetes – Answers at your fingertips** (ISBN 9781859591758)  **£17.99**

☐ **Type 2 Diabetes – Answers at your fingertips** (ISBN 9781859591765  **£17.99**

               TOTAL _____

## Easy ways to pay

**Cheque:** I enclose a cheque payable to Class Publishing for £ _____

**Credit card:** Please debit my ☐ Mastercard ☐ Visa ☐ Amex

Number _____ Expiry date _____

Name _____

My address for delivery is _____

_____

Town _____ County _____ Postcode _____

Telephone number (*in case of query*) _____

Credit card billing address if different from above _____

_____

Town _____ County _____ Postcode _____

*Class Publishing's guarantee: remember that if, for any reason, you are not satisfied with these books, we will refund all your money, without any questions asked. Prices and VAT rates may be altered for reasons beyond our control.*